Liam W

CW00435150

EAT YOURSELF SLIM

Burning fat Slimming healthily
Step by step guide
Achieve your desired weight
without renunciation

1st edition 2020

Table of contents

1. Introduction   10

2. Adequate nutrition   12

3. Eating habits over time   15

4. Health risk overweight   17

4.1 General   17

4.2 The threat of sugar   17

     4.2.1 Metabolic syndrome   18

     4.2.2 Type 2 diabetes   18

4.2.2.1 Heredity and lifestyle   19

4.2.2.2 Symptoms   20

4.2.2.3 Destroyed nerves   20

4.2.2.4 Forms of diabetes   21

     4.2.3 Is sugar addictive?   21

     4.2.4 Does sugar cause cancer?   24

4.3 Abdominal fat (visceral fat)   24

5. Slimming down correctly – working out the goal   26

5.1 What is ideal weight anyway?   28

5.2 Measuring methods healthy body weight   28

     5.2.1 Calculating BMI (Body Mass Index)   29

     5.2.2 Rating BMI (Body Mass Index)   30

     5.2.3 Calculating WHR (waist-hip quotient)   30

     5.2.4 Evaluating WHR (waist-hip quotient)   31

5.3 Define goal   32

5.4 Change the menu   33

5.5 Balanced diet   34

5.6 Why a fibre-rich diet?   35

     5.6.1 What are dietary fibres?   36

     5.6.2 What effect do dietary fibres have?   36

     5.6.3 How many grams of fibre does the body need?   37

     5.6.4 What do I need to know about dietary fibres?   37

5.7 Interval fasting and body fat reduction   37

     5.7.1 Body fat reduction   38

     5.7.2 Autophagy and ketosis   38

5.7.3 What interval fasting still achieves   39
5.7.3.1 Prevents oxidative stress and inflammation   39
5.7.3.2 Slows down the ageing process   40
5.7.3.3 Improves sleep experience   40
5.7.3.4 Improves metabolism   40
5.7.3.5 Increase in inner focus   41
5.7.3.6 Renews body cells   41
5.7.3.7 Curtails depression   41
5.7.3.8 Aids digestion and gut flora   42
5.7.3.9 Positively influences cancer diseases   42
5.8 Alkaline diet   42
5.9 Fermented food   45
   5.9.1 Overview of fermented food   46
5.10 onclusion—correct removal   49
6. Nutritional ingredients   **50**
6.1 Water   50
6.2 Carbohydrates   51
   6.2.1 good | bad carbohydrates   51
   6.2.2 Sugar | Economic factor and production   52
   6.2.3 What sugar triggers in the body   53
   6.2.4 Unmasking sugar traps | Changing shopping   54
   6.2.5 Hidden sugar in food   54
   6.2.6 Sugar alternatives   55
6.2.6.1 Honey   55
6.2.6.2 Brown sugar   55
6.2.6.3 Agave syrup   55
6.2.6.4 Coconut blossom sugar   56
6.2.6.5 Date syrup   56
6.2.6.6 Maple syrup   57
6.2.6.7 Rice syrup   57
6.2.6.8 Stevia   57
6.2.6.9 Birch sugar (xylitol)   58
6.2.6.10 Erythritol   58
6.2.6.11 Sweetener   58

6.3 Protein 61

    6.3.1 Animal protein 62

6.4 Oils | Fats 62

    6.4.1 Omega 3, 6 and 9 fatty acids 64

  6.4.1.1 Omega 3 fatty acids 64

  6.4.1.2 Omega 6 fatty acids 65

  6.4.1.3 Omega 9 fatty acids 65

  6.4.1.4 Relationship of Omega 3 to Omega 6 66

6.5 Vital substances 67

    6.5.1 Vitamins 67

    6.5.2 Minerals | Trace elements 67

    6.5.3 Secondary plant substances 68

    6.5.4 Flavour enhancers & Co. 69

7. Positive framework conditions **71**

7.1 Excursus: Water 71

7.2 Excursus: Movement 72

7.3 Excursus: Shinrin Yoku 72

7.4 Excursus: healthy intestine 73

    7.4.1 What makes the gut so unique? 73

    7.4.2 Good and bad intestinal bacteria 75

7.5 Excursus: Yoga | Meditation 76

7.6 Excursus: sleep 77

8. Negative framework conditions **78**

8.1 Noise pollution 78

8.2 Environmental toxins | plasticisers | plastics 78

8.3 Chronic stress 80

8.4 Nicotine 81

8.5 Alcohol 82

9. Dietary myths **83**

9.1 Drink at least three litres of water a day. 83

9.2 Eggs increase the cholesterol level. 83

9.3 Eating in the evening makes you fat. 83

9.4 Honey is healthier than sugar. 83

9.5 Simple sugar is worse than fructose. 83

9.6 Light products contribute to losing weight. 84

9.7 Fat makes you fat. 84

9.8 Small meals are often an advantage. 84

9.9 Fresh vegetables are better than frozen ones. 84

10. Recipes 86

10.1 Salads & Bowls 86

    10.1.1 Chickpea salad—smoked salmon strips 86

    10.1.2 Corn salad—feta cheese 87

    10.1.3 Spanish potato salad - olives - thyme 88

    10.1.4 Asparagus ham salad with couscous 88

    10.1.5 Bulgur salad with feta and beetroot 89

    10.1.6 Panzanella (Italian bread salad) 90

    10.1.7 Radish potato salad 90

    10.1.8 Asparagus salad—gnocchi—wild garlic pesto 91

    10.1.9 Orange bread salad—chicken breast fillets 92

10.2 Alkaline diet 93

    10.2.1 Oven vegetables 93

    10.2.2 Wild herb soup 93

    10.2.3 Grilled vegetables with rocket salad 94

    10.2.4 Melon Granite 95

10.3 Keto recipes 96

    10.3.1 Fried cod on courgette vegetables 96

    10.3.2 Lentil roasts 96

    10.3.3 Konjac noodles with avocadopesto 97

    10.3.4 Ketogenic almond bread 98

    10.3.5 Ricotta Quiche 98

    10.3.6 Chicken Feta Broccoli Casserole 99

    10.3.7 Radish spaghetti with vegetable bolognese 99

    10.3.8 Pan of vegetables with Thai asparagus 100

    10.3.9 Pumpkin and Spinach Curry 101

10.4 Raw food 103

    10.4.1 Gazpacho—cold tomato soup 103

    10.4.2 Asparagus Fennel Salad 103

    10.4.3 Chiapudding 104

10.5 Soups 105
    10.5.1 Pumpkin and turnip soup 105
    10.5.2 Beetroot sweet potato soup 106
    10.5.3 Thai coconut soup with rice noodles 106
    10.5.4 Apple and horseradish soup 107
    10.5.5 Curry lentil soup with baked cauliflower 108
    10.5.6 Potato and mushroom soup 109
    10.5.7 Chorizo stew 110
    10.5.8 French onion soup 111
    10.5.9 Minestrone 111
    10.5.10 Lentil soup with spinach 112
    10.5.11 Carrot soup with spelt croutons 113
    10.5.12 Parsley root soup 114
    10.5.13 Turnips Potato soup with wild garlic Pesto 115
    10.5.14 Lentil soup with chard and minced meat 116
    10.5.15 Kohlrabi Savoy Soup 117
    10.5.16 Spicy noodle soup with chicken 118
10.6 Salad dressings 120
    10.6.1 Vinaigrette, classic 120
    10.6.2 Yoghurt dressing 121
    10.6.3 Wasabi lime dressing 121
    10.6.4 Buttermilk-blackberry dressing 122
    10.6.5 Cranberry and hazelnut dressing 123
    10.6.6 Pea and balm dressing 124
    10.6.7 Mango-Jalapeño Dressing 124
    10.6.8 Blueberry pumpernickel dressing 125
10.7 Smoothie 127
    10.7.1 Chinese Cabbage Blueberry Smoothie 127
    10.7.2 Green Detox Smoothie 128
    10.7.3 Sauerkraut-Grapefruit Smoothie 129
    10.7.4 Avocado-Banana-Apple Smoothie 130
    10.7.5 Chick peas smoothie, Greek yoghurt and broccoli 130
    10.7.6 Spinach and savoy cabbage smoothie with pear 131
    10.7.7 Ginger Grape Carrot Smoothie 131

10.7.8 Pineapple-Mango Detox Smoothie 132

10.8 Healthy breakfast 134

   10.8.1 Skyr with seeds, oranges and banana 134

   10.8.2 Spelt bread with avocado cream and graved salmon 134

   10.8.3 Birch muesli with carrot boscoop salad 135

   10.8.4 Oatmeal with maple syrup and banana 136

10.9 Mediterranean 138

   10.9.1 Grilled Bread 138

   10.9.2 Fried fillet of gilthead 138

   10.9.3 Antipasti with vegetables, mushrooms and olives 140

   10.9.4 Penne in tuna tomato sauce 140

   10.9.5 Pasta salad with mozzarella 141

   10.9.6 Braised meatballs 142

10.10 Vegan dishes 144

   10.10.1 Baked aubergine and carrots 144

   10.10.2 Pak Choi with ginger-garlic sauce and sesame 145

   10.10.3 Tomatoes stuffed with oriental couscous 146

   10.10.4 Bami Goreng with broccoli and tempeh 146

   10.10.5 Sweet potato, chickpeas and almond sauce 147

   10.10.6 Courgette spaghetti with lentil bolognese 148

   10.10.7 Baked aubergine, celery puree, carrots 149

10.11 Snacks 151

   10.11.1 Leek-Paprika Muffin 151

   10.11.2 Arancini - Sicilian rice balls 152

   10.11.3 Spinach Crostini au gratin 152

10.12 Sweet reward 154

   10.12.1 Coffee Cream 154

   10.12.2 Ricotta cheesecake - hazelnut caramel 154

   10.12.3 Cheesecake Tiramisu in a glass 155

   10.12.4 Pear-Rhubarb Crumble 156

   10.12.5 Warm chocolate cake 157

   10.12.6 Semolina crème brulée with mango 158

   10.12.7 Carrots cup cake with walnuts 158

   10.12.8 Rhubarb Crumble 159

10.12.9 Low Carb cream cheese pancakes   159

10.12.10 Vanilla-Ricotta cream with blueberries   160

10.13 Baking   162

10.13.1 Best rye mixed bread without sourdough   162

10.13.2 Wholemeal spelt bread without rising   162

10.13.3 Foccacia   163

11. List of recipes   **165**

12. Conclusion   **169**

13. Feedback   **171**

14. Sources   **172**

15. Copyright   **176**

16. Disclaimer   **177**

17. Liability for links   **178**

18. Imprint   **179**

Dear reader!

I am very pleased that you have decided to buy this book and would like to go deeper into the subject of weight loss and nutrition. In this book, you will learn step by step, how it is possible to become slim in a natural way through proper nutrition and—our mutual goal—to stay slim.

Obesity is a highly topical issue that affects more and more people with each passing day. Unfortunately, more and more children and young people. In the long run, too many kilos on the ribs will make you sick. A whole series of considerable changes have an effect on our body. Overweight is not only an aesthetic problem. If we carry too much fat around with us on a permanent basis, it will lead to us having excess of inflammatory substances in our body.

Especially at the beginning, these seem like small unnoticed sources of fire. In this book I describe an understandable, everyday and varied ways to get rid of superfluous pounds.

Best regards
Liam Wade

1. Introduction

The longing for the one form of nutrition that changes everything with little effort is great. But this diet - in reality not a new insight - does not exist. According to recent studies, one in three european women regularly try out new diets. The goal: to finally reach and maintain the desired weight. But unfortunately, the truth is that only a few diets achieve permanent weight loss. Some are not only without a positive effect, but are completely questionable and can even endanger your health. Often, these are sophisticated concepts, but most of them have one basic message in common: they all divide food into good and bad. This follows people's need for simple answers to complex questions.

A change in the way we eat is needed. One sensible way to go about this is to change behaviour patterns gradually over a long period of time. Any form of nutrition that aims for quick success is doomed to failure and is dubious.

Especially in industrialised and emerging countries, the proportion of heavily overweight people is constantly increasing. In Europe, overweight is not considered a disease but a health disorder. Being severely overweight is the precursor for high blood pressure, calcification of the coronary arteries, type 2 diabetes, various forms of cancer as well as some orthopaedic and mental illnesses. The cause is usually a combination of genetic disposition and unhealthy lifestyle. High-calorie food is combined with a lack of exercise. Other factors are stress, frustration, constant availability of food, eating disorders, depression and a few medications. The initial consequences are rapid fatigue, limited mobility, problems in the spine, hips and knees and increased wear and tear on the joints—also known as arthrosis.

In this book I would like to start by showing you the risks of being overweight. After that I will show you a sensible and healthy way to lose excess pounds. Then we will look at facets of healthy eating and, we will look in detail at the main nutrients and food components. Finally, I will give you some of my favourite recipes for healthy eating and losing weight.

It will be essential for you to realise that the way we currently feed ourselves is not wanted by nature and therefore is causing us illness. Sugar and interval fasting play a primary role in our further considerations in this book.

Let's go.

2. Adequate nutrition

Statistics prove: the number of overweight people has increased dramatically in recent years. The trend is still rising. The fairytale world of healthy eating fits in with this. The term „shelf life" describes the shelf life of food and beverages, i.e. how long a product can be stored without becoming unusable, inconsumable or unfit for sale.

The price: poison in our food in the form of artificially produced flavours, antibacterial agents, colourings and preservatives. Responsible for this are hand in hand pharmaceutical and chemical companies, nutritionists with lavish contracts, unscrupulous lobbyists and politicians with the aim of creating a dream world. The advertising message: down-to-earth quality at reasonable prices produced according to grandma's recipes with local ingredients from the juicy pastures of regional farmers. But this is only fantasy. The reality is very much different.

In a very short time after the war, our food has changed more than it did in the last 20,000 years. Food production has been adapted to industrial and storage processes rather than to consumers. It was subjected solely and exclusively to the economic principle, acting rationally for a specific purpose. With given means, it has tried to put the profit in proportion to the market value of globally operating food companies. Well over 2,500 additives are permitted in our modern foodstuffs. But only just over

300 are subject to declaration. This shows an organised attack on our senses and physical integrity. Hormones and antibiotics are found in meat, antifreeze and worms in wine and ethoxyquin in fish. The food scandals of recent years have brought to light a cocktail of poisons. In the case of white sausage, the casing comes from China, the herbs from Poland and the veal from Hungary. In addition, it is rich in phosphates and flavour enhancers. 96% of broilers are fed with antibiotics. If one animal falls ill, the whole flock is vaccinated as a preventive measure—often several times. This results in 25,000 deaths per year in the European Union caused by multi-resistant germs in hospitals.

The harvest is far from sufficient to meet the demand for all the yoghurts and fruit teas. There is usually only a teaspoon of fruit in a cherry yoghurt. The taste is created by the aroma of a wood fungus. Bread rolls come as deep-frozen raw material from Asia and Africa. This list of horrors could be continued page by page. Only a few food companies provide more than 200,000 different products under an almost unmanageable number of retail chains. Three out of four foods are highly industrialised and maximised for profit.

The human evolutionary cycle of adaptation makes it impossible to adapt to this alien diet. In order to eliminate this negative development, obesity and a number of increasingly popular diseases of civilisation, this industry naturally has the appropriate products in its portfolio. Dietary products, powders for shakes, colourful and attractive packaging from the chemical building blocks of food technology.

Far from species-appropriate nutrition. Natural, fibre-rich, anti-inflammatory and nutrient-rich food would be the focus of attention. But how can our food meet these requirements when about 20% is contaminated with industrial sugar products and another 20% with white flour products? In other words, we currently cover around 40% of our food intake with empty, calorie-rich foods that contain virtually no vitamins, minerals or secondary plant substances.

3. Eating habits over time

Apart from a few exceptions, man and his ancestors have, for most of the history of development, eaten mainly or exclusively vegetable food. This is also evidenced by anatomical peculiarities such as the inability of humans to synthesise vitamin C and the lack of an enzyme that breaks down uric acid. Some researchers have even described the human dentition as that of a fructifier, and the structure of the colon also corresponds to that of a herbivore. It was only meat consumption that made the cerebrum grow.

Nowadays, a diet that is heavily based on meat can have unhealthy consequences, as our lifestyle has changed fundamentally. In the past, meat came from free-living animals whose feed did not consist of industrial waste. Food had to be hunted and earned and involved hard physical work.

Original nutrition of our ancestors[1]
- Was free from sugar.
- Was rich in secondary plant substances.
- Contained plenty of fibre.
- Was species-appropriate.
- Consisted of whole grain cereals.
- Had a balanced ratio of Omega 3 to Omega 6 fatty acids.

- Was predominantly vegetable and had few animal components.

Nutrition of today

- Has a very long list of additives such as raising agents, preservatives, colourings, synthetically produced flavours, emulsifiers, etc.
- Contains a high proportion of animal meat and sausage products, which also come from factory farming.
- Has a sugar concentration that has increased by a factor of 50 over the last 100 years in almost all industrially produced foodstuffs.
- Accepts damage to the intestinal flora caused by medication.
- Has a much too low consumption of drinking water of spring water quality.
- Means irradiation of food.
- Is a contaminated system proven by fungicides and pesticides.

4. Health risk overweight[2]

4.1 General

Too much weight puts enormous strain on the heart and blood circulation. This is because the amount of blood is greater in fat people than in people of normal weight, which means more work for the heart because it has to beat more often. High blood pressure is the consequence.

Obesity also causes long-term damage to the blood vessels throughout the body, as it encourages deposits, which ultimately leads to vascular calcification (arteriosclerosis).

Joint diseases and back problems are also direct effects of excessive weight. A person who weighs a third too much shortens his or her life expectancy by an average of three years – severely overweight people by up to ten years.

4.2 The threat of sugar

Sugar is a dose of dependent poison. One in five persons in Europe is considered to be obese. This is because the recommended amount is exceeded four times over here in Europe and causes a whole range of diseases.

4.2.1 Metabolic syndrome[3]

The metabolic syndrome is a generic term for various disorders that are caused by excessive sugar consumption. The Greek term „metabolic" means metabolically related. A syndrome is when there are different symptoms (complex symptoms) at the same time, each of which can have a different background.

4.2.2 Type 2 diabetes[4]

Every day more than 1,000 persons in Europe are diagnosed with type 2 diabetes, currently totalling more than 7.5 million. The disease is increasingly affecting younger people. Many people think they are healthy and only feel a bit flabby now and then. There can be lots of reasons why they might be ill, but only very few people ever think of that. At first, diabetes does not cause much or any discomfort, as this only happens when blood sugar is high.

If we have too much sugar in our blood, our body does not report this. The warning signal pain does not react in this case. None of those affected notice at first that a disease is imminent. Before an operation or a check-up, it is usually discovered by chance that there is an elevated sugar level and thus diabetes. Only when the blood sugar level is permanently too high do doctors speak of diabetes type 2. At the beginning of the disease, the pancreas produces too much insulin to ensure that the sugar reaches the cells after all. Doctors suspect that sooner or later the insulin-producing cells are overworked and can no longer produce insulin. Damage to the heart, kidneys, eyes and blood vessels is caused by sugar circulating continuously in the bloodstream. The risk of a stroke or heart attack is up to four times higher in people with this condition.

The cost of type 2 diabetes is estimated to be around 25 billion/year. Diabetes and secondary diseases are an enormous burden on the health care system and a major threat to the mental and physical health of those affected. Diabetes type 2 is reversible and therefore curable. Provided we reduce our sugar consumption, lose weight and get more exercise.

4.2.2.1 Heredity and lifestyle
The vast majority of people with diabetes are people with type 2 diabetes. 15%-22% of people over 65 years old have diabetes, comprising more men than women. If you go beyond the age of 70, there are more women than men.

Whether a person has type 2 diabetes depends on lifestyle and heredity. If you have a predisposition to type 2 diabetes, you can counteract the disease by taking plenty of exercise and eating appropriate food. Studies have shown that 50% of people who took the above-mentioned measures did not get diabetes. It is advisable to have your blood sugar levels checked by a doctor on a regular basis.

4.2.2.2 Symptoms

It often takes several years before type 2 diabetes is detected—the warning signs are not clear. However, there are a few signs that you might need to listen to carefully. For example, you might feel exhausted and need to sleep a lot. You are constantly thirsty and often have to go to the toilet. You lose weight for no reason. The skin on your feet is very dry.

4.2.2.3 Destroyed nerves

Type 2 diabetics are often diagnosed with a visual impairment. Many find it difficult to see at close range. If there is too much sugar in the blood, the nerves are affected. One in ten patients complain of neuropathic pain, which is nerve damage.

The fingertips start to tingle and the sensitivity of the feet diminishes. Digestive disorders often occur—some patients complain of flatulence, constipation, diarrhoea or stomach ache.

4.2.2.4 Forms of diabetes[5]

The characteristics of diabetes vary. The following is a detailed description.

Type 1: Less than 10% of diabetes patients are victims of this type. The immune system of these people is affected by a malfunction. The cells responsible for insulin have been destroyed during this process. Insulin is not produced enough. There is no cure for this type of diabetes.

Type 2: Unlike type 1, type 2 is not a disease of the immune system, but is caused by lifestyle mistakes. 90% of diabetes patients are affected. In contrast to type 1, this type is curable.

Type 3: Here you will find all types of diabetes that cannot be classified as type 1 or type 2. The cause can be a viral infection, a genetic mutation or damage to the pancreas.

4.2.3 Is sugar addictive[6]?

Clear answer: YES. Addiction does not come overnight. It usually sneaks into life unnoticed. It is not unusual to eat a piece of chocolate once in a while. At the beginning it is not a problem. Or is it?

Addiction requires a susceptible brain and other factors. Alcohol, nicotine, or in this case sugar, are the basis of addiction.

The scientific explanation: the balance of serotonin and dopamine in the brain is disturbed. If the messenger substance serotonin is too low and the dopamine level is too high at the same time, or if both substances are present in insufficient concentrations, the conditions are right for becoming addicted.

Dopamine is a largely excitatory nerve transmitter of the central nervous system and is used for communication. It is released in the brain when we are full of anticipation, for example before a romantic meeting, before a competition or before a hoped-for sense of achievement. It gives us a positive emotional experience and is also called the happiness hormone. If there is the first kiss or exceptional praise from the boss, serotonin is released. This messenger substance stands for happiness, satisfaction, relaxation and satisfaction.

If the dopamine level drops, we suffer from lack of drive and inertia. If we are moody, disappointed and worried, this has to do with serotonin deficiency and we reach for the drug sugar in such a state. This increases the levels of dopamine and serotonin and gives us a feeling of happiness and relaxation. They make us believe that we have achieved something extraordinary. That's about the scientific background.

Conclusion: Sugar acts like alcohol and nicotine, increases serotonin and dopamine levels, can be called a drug and will lead to addiction if consumed in excess. Sugar is a kind of self-delusion.

The sugar industry has long denied that there is any such thing as addiction in relation to sugar. However, there is clear scientific evidence that points to this fact. The enormous potential for addiction has been demonstrated in rats, among other animals. If rats who are used to sugar are deprived of their daily dose of sweets, they react with trembling, chattering teeth and fear. The rats then increasingly used alcohol as a substitute. When sugar was on the menu, however, they ate more than ever before. People show similar behaviour patterns.

After only a short time, changes in the brain of the rats similar to those found in chronic drug addicts were diagnosed. Drug and alcohol addicts have a conspicuous weakness for sugar products. Sugar is the number one popular drug.

4.2.4 Does sugar cause cancer[7]?

This thesis is considered to be unsubstantiated, but there are clear indications that this is the case. A Belgian research team found in a nine-year study that sugar stimulates tumour growth. In the study, the scientists observed the so-called Warburg effect over a longer period of time. This mechanism, which has been known for a long time, shows in the laboratory that cancer cells metabolise larger amounts of sugar than healthy cells.

The Canadian anthropologist Vilhjámur Stefánsson observed something astonishing at the beginning of the 20th century: Eskimos did not get cancer as long as they fed traditionally. They went hunting, kept to fixed daily rhythms, ate meat from seals, caribou or fish. It was only when they switched to carbohydrate-rich industrial food in the middle of the 20th century and became a little more comfortable that they died of cancer.

4.3 Abdominal fat (visceral fat)[8]

Visceral fat (from Latin viscera, meaning ‚the intestines'), also known as intra-abdominal fat, is the fat stored in the free abdominal cavity of vertebrates that envelops the internal organs, particularly the digestive system. 30% of people are overweight. In Europe, the figure is one in two persons. The risk of diabetes and high blood pressure increases with fat deposits around the abdominal organs.

There are two types of fatty tissue in our body. Fat on the buttocks and hips, also called subcutaneous fat tissue. It insulates, keeps warm and serves as an energy store for bad times. And it's one advantage is that it is neutral. Visceral fat is formed in the abdominal cavity and surrounds organs. Thick bellies indicate a lot of visceral fat.

Visceral fat is metabolically active, surrounds the liver and intestines, forms more than 200 hormone-like substances and is therefore one of the largest glandular organs in the body. These messenger substances have an overall negative effect on blood pressure, insulin release and inflammation. Abdominal fat is more pronounced in men. They therefore have a higher risk of contracting visceral fat. An abdominal girth of less than 94 cm is considered acceptable, in women less than 80 cm. In order to survive in bad times, our body has made it a habit to store visceral fat during stress.

5. Slimming down correctly – working out the goal

I would now like to explain to you step by step, how you can lose weight. There is no one way that suits everyone. Many questions on this subject can only be answered individually, and depend on your type and rhythm of life. The basis for losing weight is always a calorie deficit. This means that you take in fewer calories than you burn. To lose one kilo of body fat, you need to save about 7,000 kcal. To lose weight healthily and effectively, a daily calorie deficit of 300-500 kcal is recommended. You are in deficit when your body is provided with less energy than it uses. If this condition lasts longer, your body uses up its fat reserves. The answer to the question as to when to know you are in this calorie deficit is provided by your energy balance. In order to maintain this value, you need to know your energy needs, that is the calories you burn and the amount of energy you consume. That is what you should consume in the form of food and drink during the day.

Note: If your behaviour consumes more energy than you consume, you are in an energy deficit. You should therefore first calculate your calorie requirement per day, as this is the first value you need. You can do this by hand or online. If you search for the term „calorie calculator", you will quickly find it. To calculate your calorie requirement, you need information about your height, weight, age and sex. For example, for a 35-year-old woman, 170 cm tall and weighing 70 kg, who does not exercise and moves on average during work, this would be 2,200 kilocalories. If this woman consumed exactly these calories per day, she would neither gain nor lose weight. It should be noted that this type of calculation only provides average values. In order to obtain exact values, tests would have to be carried out by specialists.

In order to get an overview of your calorie intake, you should now record in detail what is on your menu. A nutrition diary will be helpful in this regard. You should keep the diet diary for a week at least before you start to look at it. You can keep a diet diary with an app on your mobile phone or tablet. If you are serious about losing weight, you will need to count a few calories.

Check the internet or your App Store to get one of these solutions. YAZIO or My FitnessPal are free of charge and good app.

If you now have both values, average calorie requirement and average calorie intake, you only need to compare them. If your calorie intake is greater than your calorie requirement, you will gain weight, and vice versa. You should be about 300-500 calories below your calorie requirement to lose weight. These values should be checked every four to six weeks, because losing weight will change them. Now all you need is your goal, and then you can start.

5.1 What is ideal weight anyway[9]?

People with a few kilos too much are often pigeonholed as „sick" and „lazy". Weight alone does not tell you anything about your state of health. Many people try to counteract the common weight norms and develop a positive relationship with their body. According to sociologists, if you are slim, you supposedly have a certain amount of capital that you can exchange for friendship, partnership or professional success. Slim people, according to sociologists, are unconsciously perceived as more trustworthy, competent, successful and healthy, unlike those whose appearance is rather below the norm. Unjust but probably human. Because we humans like things to be simple. At this point, however, we are only interested in the question of what your healthy weight can be.

5.2 Measuring methods healthy body weight

Many have an individual feel-good weight—but health risks due to too many or too few pounds on the ribs can be estimated quite accurately. Body mass index (BMI) and waist-hip-quotient (WHR) show quickly and easily whether you are normal, underweight or overweight. If you are significantly overweight, just 5% less body fat lowers blood pressure and improves sugar metabolism and blood lipid levels.

5.2.1 Calculating BMI (Body Mass Index)[10]

The Body Mass Index is the most commonly used value for assessing body weight—it helps you to better estimate your weight. It puts your body weight in relation to your height. More precisely, the body weight in kilograms is related to the height in metres squared. Important to know: The body mass index only allows a first rough estimate. For example, someone who has a lot of muscle mass can have a high BMI without being overweight in the real sense of the word. The BMI also says nothing about the distribution of body fat. In particular, too much belly fat is considered a health risk. Different rules apply to children, as they are still growing. There are special BMI tables for them.

Example: You are 1.70 metres tall and weigh 80 kilograms. Then you do the math:

1.70 x 1.70 = 2.89 Now divide your weight by this value: 80÷2.89 = 27.7

27.7—or rounded up 28—is your body mass index.

5.2.2 Rating BMI (Body Mass Index)

The ideal BMI value for women is between 19 and 24, and for men it's between 20 and 25. Statistically speaking, life expectancy is highest at this BMI value. However, the ideal BMI is also dependent on age. The BMI is by no means the measure of all things.

BMI classification of the World Health Organisation (WHO):

Category	Male	Female
Underweight	less than 20	less than 19
Normal weight	20-24.9	19-23.9
Overweight	25-29.9	24-29.9
severe overweight (grade I obesity)	30-34.9	30-34.9
Obesity grade II	35-39.9	35-39.9
Obesity grade III	40 or more	40 or more

5.2.3 Calculating WHR (waist-hip quotient)[11]

Many experts therefore consider the value „waist circumference in centimetres divided by body height in centimetres" (Waist-to-Height-Ratio, abbreviated WHtR) to be more meaningful. A value of less than 0.5 (for older people less than 0.6) is considered desirable. The waist circumference alone also helps as a rough guide: it should not exceed 102 centimetres for men and 88 centimetres for women.

5.2.4 Evaluating WHR (waist-hip quotient)

Measure the waist circumference between the lowest ribcage and the iliac crest. For the hip circumference, look for the longest stretch around your buttocks.

Example: A woman on an empty stomach has 71 cm waist circumference and 95 cm hip circumference.

The WHR is therefore: 71 cm ÷ 95 cm = 0.75

For people of average size, the waist or abdominal circumference can give an indication of existing obesity. Sports physicians classify the WHR levels (and waist circumference) of adult women and men as follows.

Women:
Normal weight WHR > 0.85 waist circumference > 80 cm
Overweight WHR < 0.85 waist circumference 80 cm to 87.9 cm
Adiposity WHR from 0.85 waist circumference over 88 cm

Men:
Normal weight WHR > 1.0 Waist circumference > 94 cm

Overweight WHR < 1.0 Waist circumference 94 cm to 101.9 cm

Adiposity WHR from 1.0 waist circumference over 102 cm

5.3 Define goal

To lose ten kilos in four weeks is a completely unrealistic goal. The human body consists of about 70% water. There are boxers who lose up to the limit of three kilos just before a competition by sweating alone, before getting into a low weight class. To store one gram of carbohydrate (glycogen), our body needs 2.7 g of water. 300-400 g of glycogen are stored in the muscle and liver. This means that another 2.5 litres of water are added. If you empty your carbohydrate stores via an extremely low-carbohydrate diet, e.g. a ketogenic diet, fasting or low carb, the body loses more water in this way. In this case, 5 kg of weight is added without even the slightest reduction in body fat. Fatty tissue is not 100% fat, but 20% water and protein, and 80% fat. So if you want to reduce 1 kg of body weight, you have to deal with 800 g fat and 200 g protein and water. So you have to save about 7,000 kcal to lose 1 kg of body fat, because 1g of fat is equivalent to 9.3 kcal. To be realistic, 250 g to 500 g body fat loss per week is possible under optimal conditions.

5.4 Change the menu

- Try to eat fresh food as much as possible and do not eat ready-made meals, which often contain sugar. Eating them is no taboo, because it must taste good. In any case, eat lots of vegetables and salad.
- Do not buy products for which advertising is made, because they are highly processed and therefore harmful in every respect.
- Avoid sweetened drinks and only drink water, tea or coffee straight. Sugar is often used as a cheap filler and flavour enhancer in ready-made foods. If you cook for yourself, you know what's in the food. Find out what suits your cooking and eating habits best and try them out.
- Getting to know and appreciate natural sweetness again—like in natural fruit, berries in particular. These have a low sugar content (about 4-8 g of carbohydrates per 100 g) and are also packed full of nutrients and antioxidants. There is nothing wrong with berries. They are even recommended because of their nutrient profile. However, it is always important to keep in check the amount consumed.

- People who start their meals with salads, vegetables and protein-rich foods, and only then switch to carbohydrate-rich foods, eat healthier. This is because the blood sugar level and thus the insulin release remain lower than if you eat the same dish in reverse order. Avoid eating carbohydrate-rich foods such as rice, potatoes, pasta, bread or even sweets on an empty stomach. It is not for nothing that a dessert is always at the end of a menu.
- Bitter substances curb appetite. Chewing the bitter calamus root is an old household remedy for ravenous appetite. You can make a tea from it. Yarrow tea works in a similar way. Chocolate with 70%-100% cocoa content tastes bitter and prevents the greed for sweets. There is also chocolate with birch sugar or erythritol. Coffee with its bitter substances is also a good appetite suppressant. In the evening, it is better to drink decaffeinated coffee.

5.5 Balanced diet[12]

The so-called Mediterranean Diet is often recommended by doctors. It was voted the best form of nutrition in 2019. The main ingredients are fish, olive oil, nuts, salad and fresh vegetables. Fatty milk and red meat in large quantities are taboo. This form of nutrition helps you to reach your desired weight. High blood pressure and cardiovascular diseases are the result of too much salt in our diet. Industrially prepared food often contains a lot of salt. Herbs such as coriander, thyme, parsley and wild garlic replace salt in the fresh kitchen. This also includes the use of garlic and onions. Sweets should be compensated for by eating nuts, which contain a high proportion of fibre and protein, as a healthy snack. Red meat is on the menu of the Mediterranean cuisine twice a week at most. Instead, poultry and fish are used as a source of protein. Milk in the high-fat version is to be replaced by the consistent use of low-fat milk. Fruit and vegetables are eaten throughout the day and are the primary ingredients. It is of central importance to take your time and enjoy it while eating, and to chew slowly. The speed at which one eats food has a considerable influence on the storage of depot fat.

5.6 Why a fibre-rich diet[13]?

Fibre stimulates digestion and prevents various diseases. Studies have shown that fibre deficiency is associated with risk factors for obesity, diabetes, high blood pressure, heart attacks and other conditions. You can lose weight tremendously with a fibre-rich diet. This is because fibre has the property of making the bowel swell. This suggests to our body that we are full and promotes the feeling of satiety.

5.6.1 What are dietary fibres?

Dietary fibres are plant fibres, swelling agents and largely indigestible food components, mostly carbohydrates, which are mainly found in plant foods. They are mainly found in cereals, fruit, vegetables, legumes and, in small quantities, in milk. For the sake of simplicity, dietary fibres are divided into water-soluble (such as locust bean gum, guar, pectin and dextrins) and water-insoluble (for example cellulose). Fibre is now considered an important part of the human diet, contrary to what the name might suggest. Their energy value is 8 KJ/g.

5.6.2 What effect do dietary fibres have?

Water-insoluble dietary fibres (such as cellulose, lignin) are source material and provide „mass". In combination with sufficient liquid, they swell up in the stomach and thus make you well-fed. They also accelerate the intestinal passage. They „clean" the intestines like a sponge.

Water-soluble dietary fibres (for example pectin, also inulin, oligofructose and other so-called prebiotics) are „bacterial food". They nourish our intestinal flora. These microorganisms are vital. They help us to utilise our food and produce healthy short-chain fatty acids.

Water-soluble dietary fibres have a positive effect on[14]:

- The sugar metabolism.
- The fat metabolism.
- The regulation of the immune defence.
- The nervous system.

Beta-glucans, soluble fibres in oats and barley, are particularly good for diabetics: they can intercept peaks in blood sugar levels and counteract insulin resistance.

5.6.3 How many grams of fibre does the body need?

You should consume between 30 g and 40 g of fibre a day. Of this, 15-20 g should come from cereals and cereal products, the rest in the form of vegetables, fruit, nuts and pulses.

5.6.4 What do I need to know about dietary fibres?

Dietary fibres swell in the intestine. This means that the intestinal volume increases significantly. In order to swell and to stimulate intestinal activity, your intestine needs fluid. The recommended amount to drink is 4% of your body weight.

5.7 Interval fasting and body fat reduction

Interval fasting is an integral part of nutritional medicine, which is considered a multi-talented method and has a number of drastic advantages.

5.7.1 Body fat reduction

Interval fasting also attacks the so-called visceral fat. This accumulates in the middle of the body and is suspected of producing and distributing hormones and inflammatory substances like an independent organ. In most people, the hormonal balance is disturbed. Each intake of calories boosts the release of insulin and thus activates the storage of nutrients. With the release of insulin, a reduction in body fat is impossible. Insulin is used in factory farming specifically to build up weight. The „hunger hormone" ghrelin is inhibited and thus ensures a feeling of satiety. Once fat has been converted into ketone, it is either consumed or excreted in the urine. Ketone bodies are not stored temporarily.

5.7.2 Autophagy and ketosis[15]

In order to live, our body needs energy, which it generates with the help of the basic building blocks contained in food. This produces valuable and not so valuable substances, some of which are harmful to humans and leave our body through detoxification processes. Autophagy is derived from the Greek word „car" for self and „phagia" for food. In 2016, the subject became more popular as the Japanese Yoshiori Ohsumi was awarded a Nobel Prize in Medicine for his research on the subject. Autophagy is our body's recycling programme, in which cellular waste is identified, recycled or excreted through the skin, lungs, blood and urine. If this programme fails, the consequences include neurodegenerative diseases such as Alzheimer's, Parkinson's, cancer or increased susceptibility to infection.

Our body has several sources that can help it to produce energy. The first source is called sugar, carbohydrates or glucose, the second is fat. Glucose is stored in the liver and muscles. This storage is empty after 24-72 hours under normal stress. Our brain depends exclusively on glucose and cannot use protein or fat. For this reason, we are able to produce alternative energy sources, the so-called ketone bodies, which are formed from fatty acids. The formation of ketone bodies from fat is possible for up to 60 days. After this time these reserves are also used up. This period of time is called ketosis or hunger metabolism. In order to reach this state outside of famine, it is necessary to reduce the intake of glucose / sugar / carbohydrates to about less than 40 g per day.

5.7.3 What interval fasting still achieves
5.7.3.1 Prevents oxidative stress and inflammation[16]

Oxidative stress is triggered by free radicals. In our body there must be harmony between oxidants and antioxidants. Free radicals are intermediate products of our metabolism. They are oxygen compounds that lack an electron. If the body does not succeed in restoring the balance, inflammations develop. Interval fasting helps you to achieve this harmony, especially by removing free radicals in times of ketosis.

5.7.3.2 Slows down the ageing process

Interval fasting slows down ageing. By lowering blood sugar, strengthening the immune system, improving cell regeneration and reducing blood pressure, the ageing process is delayed. The basis for this is autophagy and ketosis.

5.7.3.3 Improves sleep experience

Unhealthy and late eating means bad sleep. Those who eat late and especially just before going to bed get little or no rest at night. Interval fasting regulates the biorhythm and thus prevents a negative sleep experience or contributes to improvement.

5.7.3.4 Improves metabolism

The metabolism is changed from food from outside to food from inside. Interval fasting promotes the process of glycogenosis. This is the conversion from glucose to glycogen. Urea is synthesised as a by-product. This is excreted via the kidneys. Liver and kidney are relieved overall.

5.7.3.5 Increase in inner focus

The brain works better and more effectively due to the increased and altered supply of energy in ketosis. As an early remedy for epilepsy, it led to massive improvements and stabilisation of the patients.

5.7.3.6 Renews body cells

In the course of the autophagy prevailing during interval fasting, the renewal of body cells and organs is much faster and more flexible. Interval fasting controls and reprogrammes liver proteins and thus has a direct effect on liver health. The metabolism of fatty acids is also positively influenced.

5.7.3.7 Curtails depression

It has been known for some time that brief food deprivation increases tryptophan levels in the brain. L-tryptophan belongs to the 21 proteinogenic amino acids, i.e. those that are needed for the body's own protein synthesis. A low tryptophan level can lead to reduced memory performance, among other things. Various general conditions such as unhealthy nutrition or stress have a negative influence on the tryptophan level in our body.

5.7.3.8 Aids digestion and gut flora[17]

Interval fasting regulates the acid-base balance. Flour, coffee, sugary foods and alcohol, among other factors, cause the intestinal flora to be impaired and have no opportunity to regenerate. The intestine contains 80% of the immune system. Bacteria in the intestine provide metabolic products. They influence our immune system and can moderate or promote inflammatory processes.

5.7.3.9 Positively influences cancer diseases

Even if the studies are not clear, there are many indications that intermittent fasting can prevent cancer or even have a positive effect on advanced stages of the disease.

You have open questions or concerns? Just send me a mail to book_manufacture@outlook.com

5.8 Alkaline diet[18]

A whole range of health and nutrition experts consider the over-acidification of the organism to be the cause of various complaints. The acid-base balance is directly related to your health. They believe that, for example, the typically meat-heavy Western diet, which is based on an excess of animal ingredients, is responsible for more acids in the body. Basic foods such as vegetables are not consumed in sufficient quantities. There is also a lack of buffer substances such as minerals like calcium or magnesium. In this situation, our body is no longer able to excrete excess acids through the lungs, kidneys, intestines and sweat. Every cell in our body functions best within a certain pH range. This zone describes whether something is acidic, neutral or alkaline. A pH value below 7 indicates that something is acidic, while a pH value above 7 indicates that something is alkaline. Blood is in the slightly alkaline range of from 7.35 to 7.44. Many organs work best at a certain pH range. That is why people are constantly trying to maintain this ideal range and buffer and balance acids. Our body automatically deacidifies. With nutrition and a few small changes you can ensure that your balance is restored.

With these seven steps you will achieve your acid-base balance:

- Most important factor nutrition. Alkaline foods are mainly rich in minerals because they buffer the acids in the body. This includes vegetables, especially green leafy vegetables such as spinach. Herbs such as nettle or dandelion are also included. The taste of a foodstuff does not indicate whether it is metabolized to form acids or bases. The fruit acids of oranges and lemons are metabolized in our body to form bases.

- Reduce acid-forming foods to a minimum. These foods contain mainly sulphur-containing amino acids. These include meat, fish, cheese and eggs. Wholemeal products and pulses are also acidogenic, but they contain important nutrients and are good acid producers. Sweets and baked goods made from white flour should be avoided.
- Pay attention to breathing—avoid shallow breathing. The lungs are an important organ that helps with deacidification. Acids in the body are converted to carbon dioxide in the lungs and breathed out. The more intensively you breathe, the better your body is supported in the deacidification process.
- Support the liver and kidney during deacidification. Both are important organs that help your body eliminate acids. Drinking enough is the order of the day. Water enriched with lemon juice is ideal. Avoid alcohol, as it acts as a cell poison and restricts liver activity.
- If you implement more than 80% of the above advice, you have already achieved a lot. This procedure is also called alkaline excess nutrition. The remaining 20 % should be covered by good acid formers like fish.
- The skin is also deacidified. That is why regular sweating is advisable when visiting the sauna or doing sports.

- Stress should be avoided as it leads to reduced activity of the liver, kidneys and intestines. In addition, the breathing is not sufficiently deep.

5.9 Fermented food[19]

Yoghurt, cheese, kefir, wine, beer and sauerkraut. They all have one thing in common: they have been preserved by fermentation. These foods are not only easier to digest, but also keep longer. These ferments are free of preservatives and additives, healthy and tasty. Fermenting food is not a novelty.

Alcoholic and lactic acid fermentation are important. Foods are coated with a layer of salt and stored in containers under cover for a long time. This is where lactic acid bacteria develop and fermentation takes place. Fermented foods contain natural enzymes, create a positive environment in the intestines through the lactic acid bacteria when consumed, and thus strengthen our immune system. As 70% to 80% of the immune system is located in the intestine, the correct balance of the intestinal flora is important. A high vitamin content and secondary plant substances have an antioxidant, immunostimulating and anticoagulant effect. They can thus positively counteract cancer, diabetes and cardiovascular diseases. Another effect is that regular consumption of fermented food can prevent ravenous appetite, as there are fewer harmful micro-organisms in the intestines. This in turn is important to ensure that the metabolism runs smoothly and that all the nutrients that are important for the body can be absorbed.

In the late 19th century, it was observed that micro-organisms in the gastro-intestinal tract of healthy people were different from that of those who were ill. This beneficial flora was called probiotics, which literally means „for life". Probiotics are micro-organisms that have been proven to have beneficial effects on health. The reason why fermented foods and drinks are beneficial is because of the natural probiotics they contain.

Fermentation helps to produce new nutrients such as B vitamins, folic acid, riboflavin, niacin, thiamine and biotin, and has been proven to improve the availability, digestibility and quantity of some nutrients.

5.9.1 Overview of fermented food[20]

Sauerkraut

Sauerkraut is not a separate plant or cabbage genus, but rather a cabbage preserved by lactic acid fermentation. The most common types of cabbage are white cabbage and pointed cabbage. To turn cabbage into sauerkraut, all you need is a little salt and time. The rest is taken care of by the lactic acid bacteria that form on their own. The importance of sauerkraut for the diet grew especially in Central and Eastern Europe, in areas with long cold winters. People realised that sauerkraut's shelf life and high vitamin content made it ideal for protecting them from deficiency symptoms during the winter. At the same time, it could be produced and stored relatively easily and without great effort.

Yoghurt

Yoghurt originally came from the Balkans. There it was not made from cow's milk, but from goat, sheep and buffalo milk. Yoghurt has a fine, delicately sour taste, which it gets from special lactic acid bacteria. The special feature of these lactic acid bacteria is their ability to coagulate only part of the milk. The protein whey remains dissolved in the whey and is surrounded by the solid substances of the milk. This gives the yoghurt its typical, fresh taste.

Kimchi

Kimchi is a blessing for our intestinal flora. Numerous microorganisms live in it. The Korean pickled cabbage strengthens the good bacteria and stimulates digestion. The basic ingredient in most recipes is Chinese cabbage, sometimes radish. The other ingredients may vary. These include mushrooms, leek, bean sprouts, cucumber, ginger, shrimps, garlic or chilli.

The end product is a foodstuff which, in addition to its probiotic bacteria, also contains minerals, vitamins and fibre. Not without reason, Kimchi is one of the healthiest foods of all.

Kombucha

Kombucha is fermented tea. The way it is fermented makes it so special. Green tea, black tea or herbal tea (or also ginseng), special strains of bacteria, yeast fungi or the Kombucha fungus are added, which in combination with some sugar start to ferment. The resulting bioactive substances give the Kombucha its health-promoting effect.

During fermentation, a gelatinous „tea fungus"—also known as yeast or scoby—forms on the surface of the preparation liquid, the colour of which varies depending on the type of tea. The acetic acid produced during fermentation and the polyphenols it contains give Kombucha an antibacterial effect. Kombucha is healthy because a large number of secondary plant substances have an antioxidant effect on the body. Antioxidants break down free radicals, prevent cell damage and can probably even have a positive effect on liver toxicity.

5.10 onclusion—correct removal

- Stocktaking „What is—where do I want to go" based on BMI and WHR, possibly, consultation with a doctor.
- Draw up a concrete time schedule to determine the amount of reduction to be carried out, and at what time. A maximum of 250-400 g loss/week is desirable.
- Initially keep a dietary record for one week.
- Determine energy deficit—approx. 4000 Kcal per week.
- Change your diet to a predominantly fresh, fibre-rich, vegetable cuisine. Topics: basic nutrition, fermented foods, sugar under 50 g/day and only in exceptional cases. In addition, interval fasting and appropriate nutrition.
- 30 minutes of moderate sport with recovery periods at least 2-3 times per week .
- Do not put too much pressure on yourself, instead be patient.

6. Nutritional ingredients

6.1 Water

High quality water is the beginning and the basis of everything. People no longer trust the quality from the tap—and rightly so. The increasing sales of water filters prove this. Many waterworks in this country claim that water from the tap can be drunk without hesitation. The limits for harmful substances are being raised almost every year. It is a fact that drinking water contains high concentrations of pollutants such as heavy metals, pesticides, hormones, drug residues and, more recently, even sweeteners. Our body needs high-quality drinking water in large quantities to serve as a basic substance for maintaining vital functions. Pure, living water is increasingly becoming a scarce commodity. When choosing water, it is therefore important to make sure that it comes from deep springs.

Still mineral water, which is bottled in plastic bottles, tends to be contaminated. Recent studies have found pathogens for meninges, urinary tract and lung diseases. Two-thirds of all types of water sold are filled in PET bottles. Chemicals in plastics have hormone-like effects on humans. The choice of water type has a direct influence on the success or failure of your health efforts. Other functions of water: It keeps the blood fluid, serves as a coolant and is instrumental in detoxification. The recommended daily drinking quantity is 4% of body weight.

6.2 Carbohydrates
6.2.1 good | bad carbohydrates

Good carbohydrates and bad carbohydrates: Of course, it is not quite that simple. There are big differences when it comes to carbohydrates. Carbohydrates are divided into simple and complex carbohydrates. For example, if we eat a slice of bread or potatoes, a lot of insulin is released to transport the carbohydrates into the cells. Insulin, however, is responsible for the storage of abdominal fat and thus inhibits and impedes fat burning. It is important to eat foods that are rich in carbohydrates and do not raise blood sugar levels. Eating a slice of wholemeal bread with cheese has less effect on your blood sugar level than eating a slice of white bread with jam. Wholemeal products contain more fibre, which keeps you full longer and ensures a healthy digestion. Pulses, vegetables and cereals are high in fibre.

Not completely forbidden—food which you should nevertheless restrict strongly:

White Bread
White flour pasta
Potatoes
Sweets

Cakes & Biscuits
fast food
Chips
Alcohol
Juice & Lemonades

Carbohydrate-rich foods that you should eat regularly:
Oatmeal
Wholemeal pasta
Wholemeal bread
All vegetables, few potatoes
Millet
Quinoa
Nuts

6.2.2 Sugar | Economic factor and production

Sugar production is an important economic factor. 30,000 farms live from sugar beet cultivation. From October to December, harvesters pull sugar beets out of the ground. 180,000 people live from sugar production. The turnover is estimated at 20 billion euros. Corresponding lobbying work is carried out.

The Sugar Association systematically disseminates misinformation on calorie consumption, nutritional behaviour and the health consequences instead of sticking to the facts. The importance of a balanced diet is deliberately played down. For the production of white sugar, the cleaned and crushed sugar beets in high towers are associated with plenty of hot water. Milk of lime clarifies the juice, and small particles as well as floating particles can be removed. This juice contains 16%-21% sucrose. Water is then removed from the beet juice to thicken it. At this moment, so-called seed crystals are added to the mixture to allow the sugar to crystallise. Centrifugation produces white sugar crystals. This process is repeated several times until the result is white household sugar consisting of 1:1 fructose glucose. 1/8 of the sugar production goes to supermarkets. The rest goes to the industry and ends up in a long list of products such as jelly babies, chocolate, sausage, canned food and finished products.

6.2.3 What sugar triggers in the body[21]

Sugar can contribute to the development of type 2 diabetes. Normal household sugar consists of glucose and fructose. When we eat it, it is broken down. Dextrose does not take long to enter the bloodstream. The pancreas then produces the hormone insulin. This hormone acts as a door opener for fructose. It is burned in the cells and energy is produced. If we constantly take in too much sugar, we get a kind of congestion. A lot of insulin is produced, but hardly any sugar is used. Like a broken lock, the cells no longer open and close reliably over time. If the sugar remains in the blood permanently, organs and vessels are damaged.

6.2.4 Unmasking sugar traps | Changing shopping

When you visit the supermarket, try to buy products that are as fresh and seasonal as possible. Sugar serves as a cheap filler and flavour enhancer. That is why almost all ready meals contain a lot of it. As a reminder, the maximum amount of sugar recommended by the World Health Organisation is 25 g per day.

6.2.5 Hidden sugar in food[22]

The term sugar does not always appear as such in the list of ingredients, but can hide behind many terms. In addition to ingredients that have „sugar" in their name, food manufacturers also use other types of sugar or sweetening elements, some of which are difficult to recognise as sugar because of their complicated-sounding chemical name.

Manufacturers are not obliged to indicate the quantity of each type of sugar used. An orientation can be the placement of the first mentioned terms in the list of ingredients. If they are placed far in front, this indicates a high sugar content of the food. However, if different types of sugar are placed at different positions in the list of ingredients, it is often not possible to estimate the sugar content.

6.2.6 Sugar alternatives

6.2.6.1 Honey

Honey is not far from crystal sugar. Nevertheless, honey has slight advantages. It has an antibacterial effect and especially, the slightly darker varieties contain plenty of antioxidants that counteract free radicals. Interesting for allergy sufferers: by consuming local honey, one takes in pollen from the environment all year round. In many cases, this minimises irritation and reaction at flowering time.

6.2.6.2 Brown sugar

Brown sugar is hardly distinguishable from white sugar. The only difference is that a final cleaning step was omitted. Some brown syrup still sticks to the sugar crystals. There are neither advantages nor disadvantages in terms of health, but the calorie content is comparable. The only difference is that it tastes slightly like caramel and malt.

6.2.6.3 Agave syrup

Agave syrup is similar in structure to honey and is extracted from the Mexican agave plant. It consists mainly of fructose, possible side effects with high consumption are flatulence and diarrhoea. Agave syrup has a high proportion of fructose, the effects of which are known (see metabolic syndrome).

6.2.6.4 Coconut blossom sugar

The juice of the coconut palm is used to produce sugar in the greater Asia region. It is suitable for cooking, baking, and can be used in drinks. Its calorific value is comparable to that of our white household sugar. The effect on the blood sugar level is similar. It contains traces of vitamins and minerals.

6.2.6.5 Date syrup

Date syrup consists of dates, water and some lemon juice. Dates not only taste good, but are also very healthy, because dates contain not only carbohydrates and calories in the form of sugar, but also plenty of nutrients. One advantage of sweeteners that many people find interesting is that they have far fewer calories than regular household sugar. On average, there are up to 280 calories per 100 g of date syrup. For comparison: 100 g of sugar contains around 400 calories. The syrup also provides other nutrients that household sugar lacks. For example, 100 g of date syrup contains about 1.2 g protein and up to 1.4 g dietary fibre.

6.2.6.6 Maple syrup

This sweet juice comes from Canada. There the sap of the maple tree is tapped. For 1 L of syrup you need about 40 L of tree sap. The lighter the concentrate, the higher the quality. In addition, maple syrup has a number of secondary plant substances such as potassium, iron and magnesium. Nutritionally, the syrup is classified as honey.

6.2.6.7 Rice syrup

Rice honey, or rice sugar, is made by boiling rice flour with water to make syrup. Its sweetening power as well as its energy content is somewhat weaker than our household sugar. Vegans use it as an alternative to honey. As the syrup contains almost no fructose, it is suitable for people with fructose intolerance.

6.2.6.8 Stevia

Stevia is a subtropical branch species that originally comes from Paraguay and has been used there for centuries. It does not cause caries and therefore does not damage the teeth. Its sweetening power is up to 300 times stronger than our granulated sugar. Stevia is suitable for diabetics and keeps the blood sugar level constant. If you think that Stevia is a natural product, you are mistaken. The production process is highly industrialised, using environmentally harmful aluminium salts. Care should be taken when buying Stevia, as some products contain normal household sugar.

6.2.6.9 Birch sugar (xylitol)

The extraction of xylitol is based on the chemical modification of wood sugar. This occurs in nature, for example, in coconuts, corn cobs, straw and as a waste product in paper production.

Xylitol, which is used in the food industry, is a sugar substitute and, unlike ordinary household sugar, has no harmful effects on the teeth. It is similar to sugar in taste and has almost the same sweetening power. Birch sugar only metabolises little insulin and is therefore suitable for diabetics. Xylitol has a laxative effect at high intakes and is harmless in humans, but has caused severe side effects in animal experiments. In dogs, it affects blood clotting and causes serious liver damage.

6.2.6.10 Erythritol

Erythritol is completely calorie-free and therefore suitable for diabetics. It is also well tolerated and is gentle on the teeth. Unlike other sugar alcohols, erythritol does not cause flatulence, abdominal pain or diarrhoea.

6.2.6.11 Sweetener

Tastes sweet and provides almost no calories. We are talking about sweetener. They belong to the group of

„sweeteners" and have names like aspartame, saccharin or sucralose. Eleven sweeteners are authorised in Europe. In contrast to normal household sugar, they sweeten 100 to 10,000 times more. Pure sweeteners are available as small tablets, liquid and „scattered sweeteners". They are also found in a wide variety of foods, which often advertise with references such as „light", „diet" and „sugar-free". For example, fruit yoghurts, puddings, sweets, chewing gum, jams and fruit preserves can contain sweeteners. They are also used in calorie-free soft drinks.

The sweeteners authorised in Europe are considered to be safe for human health. However, recent studies suggest that sweeteners favour bad intestinal bacteria and thus damage the immune system. The European Food Safety Authority reviews all food additives before they are authorised. Experts set an acceptable daily intake (ADI) for sweeteners. ADI values are usually based on results from animal experiments. The amount that animals can ingest over a long period of time without causing adverse reactions is considered the basis. For example, if an animal can easily consume one gram of sweetener per kilogram of body weight per day, then divide this amount by 100 to be on the safe side. For humans, the ADI is then 0.01 g or 10 milligrams per kilogram of body weight. Once the sweeteners have been approved, expert panels will examine them as needed. Aspartame, for example, was suspected a few years ago to cause headaches, allergies or even cancer. The suspected links were then tested and disproved in 2013.

The following sweeteners are currently authorised in the EU:

E 950 (Acesulfame K)
E 951 (Aspartame)
E 952 (Cyclamate)
E 954 (Saccharin)
E 955 (Sucralose)
E 957 (Thaumatin)
E 959 (Neohesperidine DC)
E 960 (Steviol glycosides)
E 961 (Neotame)
E 962 (Salt of aspartame-acesulfame)
E 969 (Advantam)

The theory that sweeteners make you gain weight is based on the idea that they promote insulin secretion, which leads to cravings. The extent to which sweeteners influence sugar metabolism is still being studied. The major scientific societies agree that sweeteners are officially safe in the recommended amounts. For me, they are among the worst alternatives, as there are already studies on the risk of cancer associated with sweeteners. Sweeteners are made purely synthetically and have an indirect effect on the intestinal environment and thus on our immune system.

6.3 Protein

Vegetable protein reduces mortality Animal and vegetable protein in our food have different effects on our health. In people with existing heart disease, the consumption of animal protein has increased the mortality rate, whereas vegetable protein has a protective effect. If the energy intake of the test subjects increased by ten percent through dairy products, eggs, meat, the mortality rate through cardiovascular disease increased by eight percent. If, on the other hand, it was lowered and the proteins came from bread, pulses and pasta, the mortality rate fell. However, the link between protein consumption and mortality rates only applies to people who are living unhealthy lives overall.

Protein is found in fish, meat and eggs, but also in plant foods such as pulses and cereals. Proteins ensure lasting satiety, whereas carbohydrates promote a renewed feeling of hunger after a short time. This is why you should use vegetable protein during periods of weight loss. Protein is involved in the formation of bones and muscles. It is made up of amino acids, the smallest building blocks, and is available to your body in many variations. One gram of protein per kilogram of body weight per day is recommended. This means that a normal-weight person of 80 kg has a requirement of 80 g of protein. For older and sick people the requirement increases to 1.5 g. Different rules also apply to athletes and pregnant women. In the case of overweight, the amount is reduced by 10%.

6.3.1 Animal protein

Protein of animal origin e.g. parmesan, turkey breast, curd cheese or chicken egg, is more similar to body protein and therefore has a higher biological value. This means that the body can use it more easily to produce the body's own protein. However, vegetable protein is healthier because it contains fibre and secondary plant substances. People with kidney disease should be cautious about eating protein, because protein breakdown products can put an excessive strain on the kidneys.

6.4 Oils | Fats

Fats in food are of varying quality and account for about 35% of the total energy intake through food. A distinction is made between saturated, monounsaturated and polyunsaturated fats. In addition, fats are divided into animal and vegetable fats. Worth mentioning are so-called trans fats, which are subject to major changes by industry. Trans fats are correctly called trans fatty acids. Hardened fats such as margarine contain trans fatty acids as a component. Chemically speaking, trans fats are unsaturated fatty acids that have a double bond between two carbon atoms. They are formed during the chemical hardening of fats, are highly inflammatory and pose other risks.

Saturated fats serve our body primarily to supply energy, are mainly found in foods of animal origin (e.g. sausage or butter) and play a major role in fat metabolism disorders, as they increase cholesterol levels. According to the recommendations of nutritional physicians, saturated fatty acids should not exceed approx. 10% of daily food energy. At a reference level of 2,000 kilocalories per day, this corresponds to approximately 20 to 27 grams of saturated fatty acids.

We need **monounsaturated fats** for the functions of our cell membranes. They are particularly abundant in rapeseed and olive oil. Monounsaturated fatty acids have a positive influence on fat metabolism.

6.4.1 Omega 3, 6 and 9 fatty acids

6.4.1.1 Omega 3 fatty acids

They belong to the unsaturated compounds and are a subgroup within omega fatty acids. Omega 3 fatty acids are essential and must therefore be supplied from outside. The former name is vitamin F. The highest concentrations are found in vegetable oil: Linseed oil 56%-71%, chia oil up to approx. 64% and perilla oil approx. 60%. Perilla oil is extracted from the seeds of the perilla plant. The plant originates from East and South-East Asia and is mainly cultivated in India, China, Japan and Korea. The leading species of fish are salmon, anchovy, sardine and herring. Fishes absorb the fatty acids EPA (eicosapentaenoic acid) and DHA (docosahexaenoic acid) through their algae diet, but can also produce them themselves. The functions of DHA include protection against inflammation and infection, a healthy metabolism and support for the immune system. Furthermore, these hormones produce and regulate blood pressure. A sufficient intake of Omega 3 fatty acids through food is hardly possible. Up to 70 percent of the population is undersupplied. In contrast, the intake of unfavourable omega 6 fatty acids is disproportionately high.

6.4.1.2 Omega 6 fatty acids

Just like omega 3 fatty acids, omega 6 fatty acids fulfil important tasks in the human body. They also belong to the unsaturated essential fatty acids. These types of fatty acids not only lower the bad LDL cholesterol level, but also the good HDL levels. In addition, they are involved in the regulation of blood pressure, growth and repair processes and in the control of part of the immune defence, in the form of arachidonic acid activities. This in positive property is reversed as the intake of omega 6 fatty acids is disproportionately increased. Omega 6 fatty acids must also be supplied from outside. With today's type of nutrition, however, it is almost impossible to fall into an undersupply, as meat, safflower oil, corn oil and sunflower oil are rich in omega 6 fatty acids. A lack of omega 6 fatty acids leads to anaemia, susceptibility to infections, fatty liver and impaired wound healing.

6.4.1.3 Omega 9 fatty acids

A lack of omega 9 is unlikely because the body can produce the fatty acids itself. They are therefore not essential. Omega-9 fatty acids that can be taken in with food are erucic acid, gondoic acid, xime acid, nervonic acid and oleic acid. Oleic acid is the most important representative of this group and is found mainly in olive oil. Terms such as omega-9 fatty acids, monounsaturated fatty acids and oleic acid are often used interchangeably.

Blood lipids include LDL, HDL and triglycerides. LDL and triglycerides store fats in the blood vessels. HDL in turn breaks down the fats. An increased concentration of triglycerides and LDL cholesterol can lead to calcification and blockage of the blood vessels and thus to arteriosclerotic diseases.

Oleic acid has a positive influence on the ratio between HDL and total cholesterol, on HDL itself and on triglycerides. Fatty acid is also known as the „good cholesterol". Omega-9 fatty acids are also responsible for nerve conduction, the formation of hormones and the formation of cell membranes.

6.4.1.4 Relationship of Omega 3 to Omega 6

There is an omega-3 deficiency in our diet. Both omega-3 and omega-6 fatty acids regulate processes in the blood vessels and are involved in inflammatory processes. While omega-3 fatty acids dilate blood vessels, improve blood flow and inhibit inflammation, omega-6 fatty acids have the opposite effect. They constrict the blood vessels, promote blood clotting and have an anti-inflammatory effect. Due to an excess of omega-6 fatty acids in our modern food, omega-3 to omega-6 fatty acids are found in the ratio of 1:20 or higher. This leads to an overreaction of the immune system, permanent alert and latent inflammation. Researchers assume that our ancestors, as hunter-gatherers, had a ratio of omega-3 to omega-6 of 1:3—this is the ratio that evolution has designed our bodies for. When both fatty acids are in balance, we speak of a state that is neutral to inflammation and beneficial to health.

6.5 Vital substances

These can be divided into three main groups: Vitamins, minerals or trace elements and secondary plant substances, also called bioactive substances.

6.5.1 Vitamins

Vitamins belong to the micronutrients and are organic compounds. They are involved in almost every vital process in your body. For example, in the building of muscles or the interaction of ligaments, tendons and muscles. They also contribute to the normal functioning of the nervous system and energy balance. The majority of all vitamins are essential. This means that the body cannot produce these substances in sufficient quantities itself. That is why all essential vitamins must be taken in through food.

6.5.2 Minerals | Trace elements

Whether in metabolism, growth or blood formation, in the interaction of nerves and muscles—nothing works without minerals. For example, sodium and potassium regulate the water balance of our body. Calcium ensures strong bones and teeth. Iron is important for blood formation. And iodine maintains the function of the thyroid gland.

It is important that we are sufficiently supplied with all minerals, because no mineral can replace another. With a balanced, varied diet in the sense of the food pyramid, this is no problem.

6.5.3 Secondary plant substances

Secondary plant substances are found exclusively in plant foods. Although they are not essential to life, they mostly have health-promoting effects and are also known under the umbrella term „health-promoting substances". Secondary plant substances sometimes have very similar properties to vitamins.

So far, about 30,000 different secondary plant substances with a wide range of effects are known. Important representatives are e.g. carotenoids, glucosinolates, phytosterols and flavonoids. Secondary plant compounds are found in fruits and vegetables, pulses, (whole) grains, herbs and spices, vegetable oils, nuts, seeds, teas and coffee - and are also used in the production of food.

6.5.4 Flavour enhancers & Co.

Flavour enhancer

Glutamate is considered an indirect thickener. It causes disorders in appetite regulation and is therefore responsible for the risk of obesity and overweight. It stimulates growth control in the brain, while at the same time inducing an artificial feeling of hunger and giving foods a meaty, spicy taste. Up to one and a half million tonnes of this „spice" are produced and processed each year. It is suspected of causing diseases such as Alzheimer's, dementia and multiple sclerosis. The neurotoxic effect of this substance is believed to be responsible for the death of brain cells. Glutamate is often not declared on the packaging. The food industry often hides the dangerous powder behind terms like seasoning salt or flavour enhancer.

Our brain is normally protected against the penetration of toxic substances by the blood-brain barrier. However, some substances—including glutamate—can penetrate this natural protective mechanism.

Preservatives

More than 300 of these additives are allowed in the EU. Each substance has been tested and classified as „safe". E210-213: benzoic acid and certain salts suspected of promoting allergies.

E220: Sulphur dioxide, can cause allergic reactions, headaches and digestive problems.

E221-228: Sulphites are sulphur compounds that can cause nausea and allergies as well as asthma attacks.

E339, E340, E341, E450, E451, E452: Behind these are various phosphates. They are suspected of straining the kidneys and promoting arteriosclerosis.

Dyestuffs

To give food an intense colour, the industry has long been using natural substances as well as artificial ones. The latter in particular can be harmful to health.

E104: Quinoline yellow may promote ADHD in children.
E127: Erythrosine red can irritate the thyroid gland, additionally like E104 it can increase ADHD.
E180: Litholrubin red belongs to the azo dyes and can cause allergies.

7. Positive framework conditions

7.1 Excursus: Water

Why is water even an issue here? High quality water is the beginning of everything and therefore also the basis for losing weight. People no longer trust the quality from the tap—and rightly so. The increasing sales of water filters prove this. Many waterworks in this country claim that water from the tap can be drunk without hesitation. Nevertheless, the limits for harmful substances are being raised almost every year. It is a fact that our drinking water contains high concentrations of harmful substances such as heavy metals, pesticides, hormones and residues of pharmaceuticals. Our body needs drinking water in high quantities to serve as a basic substance for maintaining the vital functions of our body. Pure, living water is increasingly becoming a scarce commodity. When choosing water, it is therefore important to make sure that it comes from deep sources as far as possible. Still mineral waters which are filled in plastic bottles tend to be contaminated. For example, recent studies have found pathogens for meninges, urinary tract and lung diseases. Two thirds of all types of water sold in Europe are filled in PET bottles. Chemicals in plastics have hormone-like effects on humans. The choice of water type has a direct influence on success or failure in losing weight. Other functions of water: It keeps the blood fluid, serves as a coolant and plays an important role in detoxification. The recommended daily drinking quantity is 4% of body weight.

7.2 Excursus: Movement

It is a widespread misconception that you can reduce body fat with plenty of exercise. Sport is healthy and is considered a slimming tool. However, depending on body weight and muscle mass, we burn up in half an hour of swimming or jogging, but only 350 calories. And what many people don't consider: exercise in the form of sport increases appetite. Nevertheless, those who want to reduce body fat by changing their eating habits are as well advised to do regular moderate fitness training to keep their metabolism on the go and to prevent muscle mass from being lost.

7.3 Excursus: Shinrin Yoku

Shinrin Yoku comes from Japan and literally means „bathing in the forest". You don't really bathe in the forest, but you dive into the green. You do this by leaving the pace of the day behind, consciously opening your senses and letting the healing atmosphere of the forest flow through your body and mind. Deep and powerful relaxation in the here and now is the result. Trees and plants seem to produce substances that activate the autonomic nervous system and thus help to lower blood pressure. This gives our immune system a positive boost.

The more diverse the vegetation in a forest is, the more ethereal substances are in the air. According to scientific studies, movement in nature also leads to an increase in natural killer cells that seek out and destroy cancer cells. This would even contribute to long-term protection against the development of cancer.

7.4 Excursus: healthy intestine
7.4.1 What makes the gut so unique?

When it causes discomfort, that is when some people first realise how important our intestines are. In recent years it has become more and more important because it is very likely to play a central role in the development of a wide range of diseases. For more than ten years now, people have been increasingly tracking down intestinal bacteria and finding that many diseases are associated with a disturbance of the intestinal flora. It is about eight metres long and a few centimetres in diameter. More remarkable is the surface area of 30 to 40 square metres. The intestine is therefore the largest contact surface between us and the outside world. Inside the intestinal anatomy, a myriad of intestinal villi are responsible for this. Meals take up to three days to pass through the intestine. This body acts completely independently; It perceives, corrects, learns and is the seat of intuition. The enteric nervous system (ENS) enables the intestine to work independently of the central nervous system (CNS) as the only organ. The brain contains around 100 billion neurons, the number in the ENS is estimated at 100 to 200 million. The ENS is structurally and functionally similar to the brain. The intestine essentially performs two tasks. Food taken in through the mouth reaches the large intestine via the stomach and small intestine. There, vital substances are removed from the nutrient slurry and supplied to our body. For intruders such as poisons, viruses, toxins, fungi or other pathogens, the journey normally ends here in a healthy intestine. The intestine is therefore the body's largest defence and immune system. Over 70% of our immune system is located in the intestine. Several hundred billion intestinal bacteria and microorganisms have colonised our intestines. More microorganisms live in one gram of intestinal bacteria than people on earth. This intestinal flora, the constitution and composition of these bacteria are largely responsible for your wellbeing and the long-term survival of your health. The intestine in cooperation with the brain decides which food components are metabolised if, how and when. These microorganisms have a decisive influence on whether we stay healthy or are susceptible to disease. The intestine has another concern that is just as important—avoiding stress and ensuring that we get enough sleep regularly. People who sleep less than six hours on average have an increased risk of bowel cancer. Fibre-rich foods such as legumes, plenty of fresh vegetables and fruit and wholemeal products strengthen the functions of the bowel.

7.4.2 Good and bad intestinal bacteria

Our weight is also related to our intestinal bacteria, more precisely the ratio of Firmicutes to the Bacteroidetes bacteria. In people with a normal weight, the ratio of these two groups of bacteria is balanced, but in overweight people, the ratio of Firmicutes bacteria is many times higher in the intestines.

Firmicutes - „bad" intestinal bacteria

These microorganisms can split up indigestible dietary fibres from the food in a particularly beneficial way—into so-called „short-chain" carbohydrates. This produces simple sugar molecules in the intestine, which are quickly utilised by the body and immediately stored in the form of fat pads for periods of hunger. An excess supply of firmicutes means that up to 12% more calories are absorbed from each meal. Also unfavourable for losing weight is the ability of firmicutes to switch our body to economy mode during „hunger periods" and to consume as few calories as possible during fasting days. As soon as sufficient food is available again, the yo-yo effect occurs, every calorie is taken from the food.

Bacteroidetes - „good" intestinal bacteria

Today's food contains much more sugar than our body needs. Bacteroidetes bacteria recognise this diet, which is unhealthy for humans, because sugar can be quickly converted into alcohol, which in turn damages the liver. They encapsulate it directly in the intestine so that the „excess" is removed with the stool. Stool analyses show that If the intestinal flora is rich in Bacteroidetes bacteria, our excretions contain more unused calories than an excess of Firmicutes.

7.5 Excursus: Yoga | Meditation

The health care system has been recording an increase in stress-related absenteeism for some time now. Of the average 15 days of incapacity to work, just over two days are attributable to anxiety, stress disorders and depression. Every sixth child and every fifth young person shows pronounced signs of stress. What is the reason why more and more people are overwhelmed by their everyday life? Stress significantly shortens our life expectancy and increases the risks of a whole range of illnesses caused by silent inflammation such as autoimmune diseases, depression or strokes. It is always a question of the individual dose, i.e. which amount of stress is still healthy for the person in question.

7.6 Excursus: sleep

Too much or too little sleep is associated with a whole range of health problems. Research also shows that inflammation can be triggered. Sleeping at the wrong time or not enough sleep leads to numerous health problems. Too much sleep also seems to encourage inflammatory activity. It is often difficult to find out what causes inflammation. But sleep and sleep patterns seem to play a central role. Essential repairs take place in the body during sleep. Toxins and metabolic residues are removed. Hormones associated with our sleep, such as melatonin, interact with antioxidants. Due to the insufficient repair of cells, they are damaged over time, which leads to an increase in the inflammatory molecule—cytokine. In animals, sleep deprivation also leads to the release of cytokines, which in turn leads to an immune response. There is still a belief that excess sleep is beneficial to health and would inhibit inflammation. This assumption is wrong. There is a biological reason for this. Our body reacts to too much sleep with the same release of the inflammatory molecule cytokine. For most people, seven to eight hours of sleep is the right amount.

8. Negative framework conditions

8.1 Noise pollution

Unlike the eyes, the ear cannot be closed. Therefore, every sound wave and tone must be evaluated and processed by the brain. Mental illness, diabetes or sleeping problems are just some of the consequences of excessive noise exposure. Researchers have found that long-term exposure to noise from cars, trains or planes can lead to heart disease, damage to blood vessels and silent inflammation. Changes in hormone levels and other brain wave activity have been shown. Stress hormones have been released, sleep is affected and high blood pressure and heart attacks can occur as a result of this exposure.

8.2 Environmental toxins | plasticisers | plastics
Environmental toxins

Eight million people in developing and emerging countries die every year as a result of contact with contaminated air, water or soil. Toxins are just as common everywhere in Europe—from air and food to furniture or drinking water. It seems impossible to completely avoid contact with toxins. But you can raise your awareness to reduce the impact to a minimum. Highly dangerous pesticides are a cause of health and environmental damage worldwide, with massive consequences for the integrity of people. The most harmful environmental toxins include mercury, hexavalent chromium, radionuclides, pesticides and cadmium.

Plasticizer

Plasticizers (phthalates) are a group of industrial chemicals that give flexibility and strength to consumer and construction products, particularly those made of polyvinyl chloride (PVC) or vinyl plastic. About 90% of plasticisers are used in vinyl and are widely used. They can leach, migrate, evaporate and accumulate in household dust. Many softeners affect the male sex hormone through their hormone-like effect. A disruption in testosterone activity, especially at the beginning of life, can have irreversible effects on male reproduction. Infertility, reduced sperm count and testicular atrophy have been demonstrated in male animals.

Plastic

Plastic food containers are full of harmful chemicals. Plastics are made from refined crude oil and contain chemicals such as BPA (bisphenol-A), which act mainly as plasticizers to make plastic more durable and flexible. While these make plastic suitable for everyday use, they pose a significant risk to health, especially when they come into contact with food.

When plastic containers are used for storage or heating, chemicals can move from the containers into the food. Studies have shown that high doses of BPA cause a number of serious health problems such as diabetes, heart disease and liver damage. To (supposedly) solve this problem, companies have started to produce plastic that is labelled „BPA-free". In these products BPA is replaced by other chemicals, BPS (Bisphenol-S) and phthalates such as diethylhexyl phthalate (DEHP). However, in many cases the health risks remain. In particular, the chemicals in BPA act in a similar way to oestrogen and in the long term can have a lasting effect on women's hormone balance and can have a negative impact on reproduction. Research has linked BPA to breast cancer in animals, along with obesity, thyroid problems and neurological disorders in humans. Contact with high concentrations of phthalates and BPA during pregnancy causes lung problems in children, which often lead to chronic asthma later on. Increased insulin resistance and high blood pressure can also be observed in children.

8.3 Chronic stress

Stres is a constant and ever-present aggressor that attacks every tissue, especially the walls of arteries. Primarily a nervous system, stress affects the whole organism. The inflammations it causes develop silently without the need for infection or germ contamination.

Vascular constrictions and the associated diseases such as angina pectoris, stroke or heart attack are the result. The human being associates stress with flight and struggle. Thousands of years old evolutionary mechanisms that have been adopted 1:1 into modern times are taking effect. In order to survive these situations, the body must be provided with energy. Stress systems are activated. This begins in the brain. Neurotransmitters ensure the release of rapid energy in the form of sugar. At this point, the signs of flight and struggle are present. This leads to insulin release, which in turn can lead to a renewed craving for sugar. To end this cycle, it is advisable to reduce stress levels, e.g. through meditation or exercise, and to eat food that requires as little insulin as possible for metabolism. In this situation, exercise is usually not necessary, but it is a way to reduce stress and cortisol concentration in our body.

8.4 Nicotine

Inflammatory processes in the mouth are triggered by smoking and make wound healing more difficult. The harmful substances contained in tobacco smoke increase the inflammatory potential by a factor of 2-6, they constrict the blood vessels and thus disrupt the blood supply in the event of inflammation. Nicotine promotes the development of chronic inflammation and is therefore the precursor of many diseases, especially cancer. Tobacco is considered the main cause of cancer and the polycyclic hydrocarbons and nitrosamines it contains are highly pro-inflammatory and carcinogenic.

8.5 Alcohol

Alcohol damages all organ systems. Persistent alcohol consumption leads to inflammation of the liver. Alcohol is often the cause of inflammation of the pancreas (pancreatitis) and stomach lining (gastritis). Even the smallest amounts of alcohol attack the mucous membrane cells in the mouth, oesophagus and stomach. The likelihood of heart muscle disease and high blood pressure is significantly increased by alcohol.

9. Dietary myths

9.1 Drink at least three litres of water a day.

This assumption is wrong. Drinking should be 4% of body weight. Which would mean 3.4 litres for an average person weighing 85 kilos.

9.2 Eggs increase the cholesterol level.

The body regulates the absorption of cholesterol and excretes excess. We need this fat-like substance to stay alive.

9.3 Eating in the evening makes you fat.

It is not the time but the amount of energy that determines whether depot fat is created.

9.4 Honey is healthier than sugar.

Honey contains minute amounts of antioxidants, so it is considered a miracle cure for coughs and diabetes. This is not the case, because the other ingredients in honey are negligible. The water content is 20%.

9.5 Simple sugar is worse than fructose.

Fruit sugar (fructose) is found in fruit, among other things. The assumption that fructose has fewer calories than simple sugar is wrong. However, you should not do without the moderate consumption of fruit, because it contains other valuable components. In apples, for example, pectin.

9.6 Light products contribute to losing weight.
Light products contain less fat, but more simple sugars to compensate for the supposed lack of taste. By assuming that light products would have a positive effect on a change of diet, more is eaten.

9.7 Fat makes you fat.
The opposite is the case. Fat has twice as much energy as sugar or protein. However, this alone cannot lead to the assumption that the consumption of excessive fat leads to weight gain. Special fats, such as MCT coconut fat, contribute to the faster achievement of ketosis.

9.8 Small meals are often an advantage.
Many small meals reduce insulin sensitivity. This results in abdominal fat. The assumption that smaller meals would boost the metabolism is wrong. Our body does not care how many times a day we eat.

9.9 Fresh vegetables are better than frozen ones.
Incorrectly stored vegetables and fruit lose significant amounts of vitamins within a few hours. Frozen vegetables contain more vitamin C than comparable fresh vegetables from the retailer. Frozen blueberries regularly

receive top marks in blind tastings compared to fresh blueberries in terms of taste.

10. Recipes

The quantities in the recipes are expressed in grams (g). Millilitre (ml) corresponds to gram (g). In the case of any deviation, this will be mentioned separately. In most recipes sugar has been replaced by erythritol. Erythritol looks very similar to the classic sugar. According to the Deutsche Apothekerzeitung, it has about 70 percent of the sweetening power of sugar, so you need to dose erythritol a little higher when sweetening. This sugar substitute is suitable for cooking and baking. Erythritol has no effect on blood sugar and insulin levels, so diabetics can easily use erythritol. What is special about erythritol is that it is natural, because it is produced during the fermentation of mushrooms and occurs naturally, for example in pears, melons and grapes.

10.1 Salads & Bowls

10.1.1 Chickpea salad—smoked salmon strips
You need:

500 g of pre-cooked chick peas, half a skin of cherry tomatoes, two spring onions, 100 g of smoked salmon, two shallots, half a bunch of leaf parsley, 30 g of olive oil, juice and skin of one lemon, salt, pepper, two red peppers, half a bunch of fresh mint.

And here's how it works:

Pour the chickpeas through a sieve and rinse several times. Halve the cherry tomatoes and marinate them with salt, pepper and a little erythritol. Clean the spring onions and cut into fine strips. Do the same with the shallots. Wash the leaf parsley, dab dry and chop finely. Halve the peppers, remove the core and cut into fine strips. Mix everything together in a bowl. Arrange the salad and garnish with the smoked salmon strips.

10.1.2 Corn salad—feta cheese

You need:

One kilo of panicle tomatoes, 300 g of feta cheese, 200 g of canned corn, 100 g of kenya beans, two medium sized onions, 30 g of paprika powder sweet, a clove of garlic, 30 g of olive oil, salt, pepper.

And here's how it works:

Wash the tomatoes, remove the stalk and cut into large pieces. Pour the corn and kenya beans through a sieve and wash them carefully with lukewarm water. Cut the cheese into large pieces. Peel the onions and cut into fine strips. Peel and finely chop the garlic. Mix everything together in a bowl and season with paprika powder, olive oil, salt and pepper.

Feta cheese is a brine cheese originally made from sheep or goat cheese. It gets its spicy taste from maturing in a brine.

10.1.3 Spanish potato salad - olives - thyme

You need:

One kilo potatoes, three cloves of garlic, two shallots, 20 g of olive oil, salt, pepper, half a bunch of fresh thyme, 40 g of dried tomatoes, half a bunch of leaf parsley, 40 g of green olives without stones

And here's how it works:

Peel the potatoes and cut into cubes of about 3 cm. Cook the potatoes in salted water until they are not soft but firm to the bite. Soak the dried tomatoes in some water for half an hour. Then drain the potatoes and fry them in some olive oil until it turns golden brown, season lightly with salt. Peel the garlic and cut into fine cubes. Peel the shallots and cut into fine strips. Wash and finely chop the parsley. Pluck the thyme. Drain the olives and cut into strips. Mix everything together in a bowl and season with salt and pepper.

The essential oil of thyme, called thymol, inhibits the growth of bacteria and viruses and is therefore one of the most important remedies for coughs, colds and bronchitis.

10.1.4 Asparagus ham salad with couscous

You need:

200 g of white asparagus, 200 g of green asparagus, 100 g of couscous, 50 g of baby spinach, 30 g of olive oil, salt,

pepper, erythritol, 30 g of white wine vinegar. 100 g of Parma ham.

And here's how it works:
Peel the white asparagus and cut it into pieces about 3 cm long. Cut the end of the green asparagus about 2 cm long. Young green asparagus does not need to be peeled. Lightly roast the asparagus together in a pan, add a little water, season with salt, pepper and erythritol. When still warm, mix with the vinegar. Cook the couscous according to the instructions. Wash baby spinach and dry it with a kitchen towel. Mix all ingredients, season with salt and pepper and garnish with Parma ham.

10.1.5 Bulgur salad with feta and beetroot

You need:
110 g of bulgur, 20 g of dill, 10g of parsley, 30g of cherry tomatoes, 110 g of yoghurt, two eggs, 40 g of feta, 30g of whole hazelnuts, 140 g of cooked beetroot, half a lemon, garlic, olive oil, salt, pepper.

And here's how it works:
Pour the same amount of hot water over the Bulgur. Salt lightly and leave to swell for 15 minutes. Stir occasionally. Wash and chop the dill and parsley. Boil the eggs hard for 13 minutes. Then peel and roughly dice them. Dice the feta cheese. Roast the hazelnut kernels without fat in a hot pan. Then cut into coarse pieces. Cut the beetroot into cubes of about 3 cm. Clean the garlic and cut into

cubes. Season everything with salt, pepper, olive oil and garlic. Carefully mix all ingredients and put them into a suitable container, for example preserving jars.

Beetroot contains betaine and the B-vitamin folate, which together lower blood cholesterol levels. The effect of the tuber can prevent arterial diseases and heart disease.

10.1.6 Panzanella (Italian bread salad)
You need:
A stick of Chiabatta bread, preferably from the previous day, 500 g of panicles of tomatoes, three shallots, two cloves of garlic, 30 g of erythritol, 30 g of olive oil, salt, pepper, a fresh pot of green basil, white wine vinegar.
And here's how it works:
Coarsely dice the chiabatta bread and toast it in a pan with olive oil. Wash the tomatoes, remove the stalk and cut into slices. Coarsely pluck the basil. Clean and slice the shallots and garlic. Mix all the ingredients in a bowl and season to taste with a little olive oil and white wine vinegar, salt and pepper.

10.1.7 Radish potato salad
You need:
600g of waxy potatoes, 1 bunch of radishes, 4 shallots, 1 bunch of chives, 200 ml of vegetable stock. 1 teaspoon of mustard, 60 ml of apple vinegar, 20 ml of wheat germ oil.

And here's how it works:
Clean the potatoes and cook them unpeeled in salted water until al dente. Peel the potatoes warm. Heat vegetable stock and add mustard and vinegar. Cut the jacket potatoes into thin slices when cold. Pour the boiling vegetable stock over the potatoes and stir carefully. Wash the radishes and use a slicer to make fine slices. Add the radishes to the potatoes and then refine with sprouting oil.

10.1.8 Asparagus salad—gnocchi—wild garlic pesto

You need:
450 g of white asparagus, 390 g of gnocchi, 100 g of olive oil, 50 g of wild garlic, 20 g of parsley, 110 g of young leaf spinach, two teaspoons honey, two tablespoons pine nuts, 40 g of grated Parmesan cheese, salt, pepper, 30 g of white wine vinegar.

And here's how it works:
Peel the asparagus and cook in salt and sugar water until al dente. Then take them out and let them cool down. Wash the spinach thoroughly. Cut the asparagus into 8 cm long pieces. Fry them in a pan with the gnocchi. Wash the parsley and wild garlic. Roast the pine nuts without fat in a pan. Make a pesto with the honey, pine nuts, parmesan, salt and pepper in a mixer. Mix the asparagus together with the gnocchi and spinach in a bowl with the vinegar and arrange on a plate.

Asparagus contains vitamin C, vitamin E and the B vitamins which are important for the nervous system. Asparagus contains aspartic acid as a special ingredient. It stimulates kidney function and thus has a draining effect. If you suffer from dropsy or are overweight, it is advisable to eat asparagus.

10.1.9 Orange bread salad—chicken breast fillets

You need:

Two medium-sized shallots, half a bunch of leaf parsley, 30 g of agave syrup, salt, pepper, 30 g of olive oil, half a stick of baguette bread, five medium-sized oranges, 150 g of chicken breast fillet.

And here's how it works:

Cut the baguette bread into approx. 4 cm large rough cubes. Fry in a pan with olive oil. Cut the chicken breast fillets into thin strips and fry them in some oil. Season with salt and pepper and drain on a kitchen roll. Peel and fillet the oranges. Peel the shallots and cut into fine cubes. Wash the leaf parsley, dab dry and cut finely. Mix everything in a bowl.

10.2 Alkaline diet

10.2.1 Oven vegetables

You need:

300g of aubergine, 300 g of courgettes, 300 g of brown mushrooms, 300 g of yellow and red peppers, 3 red onions, 4 cloves of garlic, 50 g of olive oil, rock salt, pepper, 3 sprigs of rosemary.

And here's how it works:

Wash and clean all vegetables. Cut the aubergine and courgette into 2 cm thick slices. Cut the bell peppers into thick strips, peel the red onion and quarter it. Do not wash the mushrooms, just clean them. Mushrooms behave like sponges and lose a lot of flavour and consistency when washed. Mix all the vegetables very well in a large bowl with salt, pepper, olive oil, garlic and the rosemary and cook on a baking tray at 180 degrees for about 40 minutes.

10.2.2 Wild herb soup

You need:

300g of wild herbs (e.g. dandelion, wild garlic, sorrel), 120 g of leek, 80 g of celery, 100 g of carrots, 2 shallots, salt, pepper, 100 ml of cream, 80 g of butter, 40 g of spelt flour.

And here's how it works:

Wash and clean the vegetables and cut into large cubes. Wash wild herbs and dry with a kitchen towel. Heat 40 g of butter in a pot and sauté the cleaned vegetables in it. Add 500 ml of water and the cream. Season with salt and pepper. Knead the rest of the butter with the spelt flour. Cook the vegetables for about 15 minutes and puree them with a hand blender. Add the flour butter and seduce with a whisk. Cook for another five minutes. Separate the wild herbs finely. Put a small part aside for decoration. Add the remaining part to the soup and puree with a hand blender. Serve on preheated plates and decorate with the remaining wild herbs.

10.2.3 Grilled vegetables with rocket salad

You need:

190 g of mushrooms, 210 g of carrots, 220 g of courgettes, 1,800 g of aubergines, 200 g of pickled artichokes, 200 g of shallots, 450 g of dark Aceto Balsamico, 180g of erythritol, salt, pepper, three cloves of garlic, 140 g of olive oil, 310 g of rocket, 200 g of Parma ham, sliced.

And here's how it works:

Wash and clean the vegetables and cut them into pens. Cut large mushrooms in half. Sauté the vegetables one after the other in olive oil, season with erythritol, add vinegar and vegetable stock. Let the vegetables cool down, store them separately and season with salt, pepper and garlic. Arrange grilled vegetables alternately with rocket and Parma ham in large glasses or suitable containers.

10.2.4 Melon Granite

You need:

1/4 of watermelon, juice and peel of two limes, 30g of agave juice.

And here's how it works:

Clean the watermelon and put only the pure fruit flesh in a blender jug. Wash the limes, grate the peel. Finely puree them all together with the agave syrup and freeze them on a flat baking tray. From time to time, use a spatula to loosen the already frozen ice from the tray until an ice cream mass is formed.

10.3 Keto recipes

10.3.1 Fried cod on courgette vegetables

You need:

400 g of cod fillet, salt, pepper, juice of half a lemon, 400 g of courgette vegetables, a vine tomato, 10 g of red curry paste, 20 g of olive oil.

And here's how it works:

Clean and wash the courgette and then cut them into sticks of about 5-7 cm. Drain the cod on a kitchen towel and season with salt, pepper and the juice of the lemon. Wash the vine tomato, remove the greenery and cut into fine cubes. Sauté the cod in olive oil and cook in an oven at 120°C. Fry the courgette vegetables in olive oil until very brown, add the diced tomatoes, season with salt, pepper and the red curry paste. Arrange the courgette and tomato sticks on a preheated plate and place the cod on top.

10.3.2 Lentil roasts

You need:

190 g of lentils, 110 g of onions, 100 g of leeks, 100 g of carrots, 100 g of mushrooms, four tablespoons of coconut flour, a teaspoon of curry, salt, pepper, 40 g of olive oil, a small red medium hot chilli pepper.

And here's how it works:

Soak the lenses overnight. Clean or wash the onions, carrots, leeks and mushrooms and then chop them up. Pour lentils through a sieve and drain. Clean and chop the chilli pepper. Mix all ingredients in a food processor with a fast rotating knife to a homogenous mass. Heat the olive oil in a pan and arrange evenly shaped lentil roasts on both sides.

10.3.3 Konjac noodles with avocadopesto
You need:
500 g of konjac noodles, two avocadoes, 100 g of dried tomatoes, two cloves of garlic, 90 g of pine nuts, half a pot of basil, 40 g of olive oil, salt, pepper.

And here's how it works:
Roast the pine nuts without fat in a pan. Soak the tomatoes in lukewarm water for half an hour. Remove the flesh from the avocado. Squeeze the tomatoes. Pluck the basil. Mix all the ingredients except the pasta using a hand blender to make an avocado-basil pesto. Cook the konjac noodles according to the instructions and fold in the avocadopesto.

Konjac noodles are particularly popular in Chinese and Japanese cuisine. They are made from the konjac root and have almost no calorific value.

10.3.4 Ketogenic almond bread

You need:

310 g of almond flour, 260 g of linseed flour, 4 eggs, 40 g of coconut flour, half a cube of fresh yeast, 1 teaspoon of sugar, 1 teaspoon of salt.

And that's how it works:

Mix all ingredients and work into a homogenous dough. Cover and leave to rise in a warm place for 60 minutes. After 60 minutes knead and leave to rise for a further 60 minutes. Preheat an oven to 180 degrees. Line a box form with baking paper and bake the dough in it for about 55 minutes. The sugar contained in the dough has been added to loosen it up and „as food" for the yeast and is no longer present at the end of the baking process.

10.3.5 Ricotta Quiche

You need:

40 g of linseed flour, 10 g of coconut flour, 40 g of almond flour, 10 g of chia seeds, 3 g of psyllium husks, 80 ml of water, salt, 410g of ricotta, a bunch of basil, a clove of garlic, three spring onions, four eggs, 100 g of grated Parmesan cheese, 50 ml of lemon juice, salt, pepper.

And here's how it works:

Knead psyllium husks, chia seeds, coconut flour, almond flour, linseed flour, salt and water to a dough.

Clean and slice the spring onions. Mix the ricotta together with the chopped basil, crushed garlic clove, spring onions, eggs, parmesan, lemon juice, salt and pepper. Roll out the dough and line an ovenproof dish with it. Pour in the ricotta cream and bake at 180°C for 35 minutes.

10.3.6 Chicken Feta Broccoli Casserole

You need:

360 g of chicken breast fillet, 100 g of feta cheese, 200 g of cream, 50 g of pesto, salt, pepper, 150 g of broccoli, 30 g olive oil, 120 g of grated Emmental cheese, 20 g of chopped garlic, one small red chilli pepper chopped.

And here's how it works:

Cut the chicken breast fillets into approx. 5 cm pieces. Cut the broccoli into florets and cook in slightly salted water for about 5 minutes. Heat 20 g of olive oil in a pan and brown the chicken breast fillets in it. Season with salt and pepper. Dice the feta cheese. Mix all ingredients, season with salt and pepper and bake in an ovenproof dish at 180°C for approx. 45 minutes.

10.3.7 Radish spaghetti with vegetable bolognese

You need:

200 g of carrots, 200 g of courgettes, 200 g of celeriac, one red pepper, six shallots, two cloves of garlic, two small red medium hot chillies, 200 g of canned peeled tomatoes, 60 g of olive oil, salt, pepper, three tablespoons tomato puree, 250 ml of red wine, half a bunch of leaf parsley, 600 g of white radish.

And here's how it works:

Wash the carrots, celery, courgette, peppers and shallots and cut into fine cubes. Heat olive oil in a medium pot and steam the vegetables for about two to three minutes at medium heat. Add tomato paste and steam for another two minutes. Deglaze with red wine and boil down strongly. Add peeled tomatoes, bring to the boil and season with salt and pepper. Cook for another 30 minutes.

Clean the radish and turn it over a spiral slicer. Heat olive oil in a suitable pan and warm the radish over a high heat. Season with salt and pepper.

Arrange the radish noodles on preheated plates together with the vegetable bolognese.

10.3.8 Pan of vegetables with Thai asparagus

You need:

450 g of white asparagus, four shallots, two red peppers, 100 g of fresh bamboo shoots, 100 g of fresh mung bean sprouts, 40 ml of rapeseed oil, 30 ml of soy sauce, 30 ml of teriyaki sauce, 20 g of ginger, two cloves of garlic, a stick of lemon grass, a small medium hot pepper, 200 ml of coconut milk, salt, pepper.

And here's how it works:

Peel the asparagus and cut into pieces of about 5 cm. Clean the shallots and cut them into pieces. Halve the peppers and cut them into large pieces. Clean ginger and garlic and cut into fine pieces. Heat rapeseed oil in a frying pan. Steam asparagus, peppers, shallots, bamboo shoots, mung bean sprouts well. Add lemongrass. Deglaze with coconut milk, teriyaki sauce and soy sauce. Reduce slightly, remove lemongrass. Arrange the vegetable pan on preheated plates.

The word „Teriyaki" is based on the Japanese words „teri" for shine and „Yku" for grilling or braising. Teriyaki sauce is mostly made from soy sauce, rice wine, honey and spices.

10.3.9 Pumpkin and Spinach Curry

You need:
300 g of Butternut pumpkin, 400 g of fresh leaf spinach, 4 shallots, 30 g of fresh ginger, 2 small medium hot red chillies. 1 teaspoon of cumin, 2 cloves of garlic, 30 g of rape seed oil, 200 ml of coconut milk, 200 g of vegetable stock, salt, pepper, juice and zest of one lemon, 10 g of hot curry powder.

And here's how it works:
Peel the pumpkin, remove the seeds and dice the flesh. Wash the spinach and remove thick stalks. Peel and grate the ginger. Clean garlic and chop finely. Clean the chilli pepper and cut into small cubes. Peel and chop the shallots.

Heat the oil and fry pumpkin, shallots, curry powder, ginger, cumin, garlic and chilli for about one minute. Add vegetable stock and coconut milk and cook for about 20 minutes until the pumpkin is cooked. Add the spinach and work through briefly until the spinach has collapsed. Add salt, pepper and lemon juice to taste.

10.4 Raw food

10.4.1 Gazpacho—cold tomato soup

You need:

A kilo of vine tomatoes, half a stick of celery, a cucumber, three slices of toast, a clove of garlic, a red pepper, three tablespoons of red wine vinegar, two medium shallots, olive oil, salt, erythritol, half a pot of basil, pepper.

And here's how it works:

Remove the crust from the bread and soak in cold water. Wash the tomatoes, remove the greenery and cut into large cubes. Wash and finely dice the celery with the cucumber and pepper. Squeeze the soaked bread and puree it together with the tomatoes, garlic, salt, erythritol, pepper and water with a hand blender. Mix the remaining vegetables with the pureed tomatoes and season with salt, erythritol, pepper, vinegar and basil.

Gazpacho is a traditional Andalusian soup and is served as cold soup on hot days.

.

10.4.2 Asparagus Fennel Salad

You need:

A tuber of fennel, 30 asparagus spears, 2 avocados, juice and peel of a lemon, two tablespoons of linseed oil, salt, pepper, two tomatoes.

And here's how it works:

Brush and clean the fennel in water. Cut the avocados in half, remove the seeds and cut into cubes of approx. 2 cm thickness. Peel the asparagus. Use an Asian slicer to slice fine strips and do the same with the fennel bulb. Wash the tomatoes and cut into fine cubes. Mix all ingredients in a large bowl. Season to taste with salt, pepper, erythritol and lemon juice as well as linseed oil and leave to stand for an hour. Serve cold. Linseed oil seeds have a high content of alpha linolenic acid, which is one of the omega-3 fatty acids. These have an anti-inflammatory effect and regulate blood lipids, which in turn can have a positive effect on thrombosis, strokes and heart attacks.

10.4.3 Chiapudding

You need:

15 tablespoons of chia seeds, 500 g of water, a teaspoon of cocoa, 20 g of sunflower seeds, 200 g of blueberries, two tablespoons honey.

And here's how it works:

Let the chia seeds soak in water overnight. Mix the berries together with the honey using a hand blender to make a puree. Roast the sunflower seeds without fat in a pan. In tall glasses, first layer the chia seeds, then the berries. Garnish with cocoa and sunflower seeds.

Chia is a pseudo grain cultivated by the Mayas and Aztecs. The fruits of this ornamental plant come from Central America. Chia seeds are considered to be extremely healthy and can be used in smoothie, soup or salad.

10.5 Soups

10.5.1 Pumpkin and turnip soup

You need:

360 g of pumpkin, 300 g of turnips, an onion, a clove of garlic, a red pepper, a bunch of spring leek, 800 g of vegetable stock, 40 g of rapeseed oil, 10 g of paprika powder, 10 g of curry powder, 10 g of chilli powder, salt, erythritol, pepper, 40 g of white wine vinegar.

And here's how it works:

Wash the pumpkin, remove the skin and cut into pieces of about 2 cm. Do the same with the turnips. Clean and chop the onions and pepper. Heat the pumpkin, turnips and onion in a medium pot together with the rapeseed oil and sauté the vegetables until they have taken on some colour. Fill up with the vegetable stock. Cook the soup for about 20 minutes. Flavour slightly sweet and hot with salt, erythritol, pepper, white wine vinegar, powder and paprika powder.

Pumpkin shows its effects in cardiovascular diseases and high blood pressure. Carotenoids and fibre reduce the risk of cardiovascular diseases. The potassium content strengthens the heart as it protects against high blood pressure.

10.5.2 Beetroot sweet potato soup

You need:

130 g of sweet potatoes, 200 g of pre-cooked beetroot, 130 g of waxy potatoes, one medium onion, 20 g of butter, one orange, 30 g of ginger, 10g of garlic, one litre of water, curry powder, coriander, paprika powder, turmeric, 100 g of pre-cooked chickpeas, 150 g of cream, one litre of vegetable stock.

And here's how it works:

Peel the sweet potatoes and cut into cubes of about 1 cm. Drain the beetroot and cut into cubes. Peel and dice the potatoes. Clean and chop the onion. Grate orange peel and squeeze orange. Clean ginger and garlic and chop finely. Sweat sweet potatoes, potatoes, onions, ginger, garlic in a little butter. Fill up with vegetable stock. Add chick peas. Puree with a blender for about 5 seconds. Add the cream. Bring to the boil and season to taste with curry powder, coriander, paprika powder, turmeric, salt and pepper.

10.5.3 Thai coconut soup with rice noodles

You need:

100 g of shiitake mushrooms, 100 g of baby spinach, two tablespoons of lime juice, two teaspoons of lime zest, two spring onions, two medium sized carrots, 500 g of coconut milk, a bunch of fresh coriander, 210 g of rice

ribbon noodles, 45 g of red curry paste, kafir lime leaf, 20 g of rape seed oil, salt, pepper, 100 g of peanuts.

And here's how it works:

Clean the mushrooms and cut into fine strips. Brush the carrot under water and peel into fine strips with a peeler. Wash the coriander and pluck finely. Grate the lime, then halve and juice it. Heat the oil and fry the curry paste lightly for one minute. Add milk and 450g of water and bring to the boil briefly. Add the pasta. Add spring onions, carrot strips, mushrooms, kafir lime leaf, lime juice and lime zest and cook for 5-6 minutes. Remove the kafir leaf and add the spinach. Bring to the boil once briefly and then serve the soup immediately. Decorate with chopped peanuts and coriander.

Kafir limes are cultivated exclusively as spice and medicinal plants and have an intense lemon flavour. The leaves are said to have antioxidant, antibacterial and anti-inflammatory properties.

10.5.4 Apple and horseradish soup

You need:

Four large boscoo apples, a fresh horseradish, 30 g of butter, 200 g of white wine, 400 g of vegetable stock, 100 g of cream, salt, pepper, lemon juice, a medium-sized shallot, 30 g of rapeseed oil, a small medium hot chilli pepper, a small bunch of chervil.

And here's how it works:

Wash the apples but do not peel them, cut them into quarters, remove the core and cut one apple into cubes and set aside. Grate the horseradish with a peeler and then with a grater. Sauté the apple cubes in butter and season with some erythritol. Clean the shallot and cut into cubes. Do the same with the chilli pepper. Heat rapeseed oil, sauté the shallots and apple cubes for one minute. Wash the chervil, pluck and put aside. Top up with vegetable stock, white wine and cream. Bring to the boil and leave to stand for five minutes. Use a blender to thicken the soup and then season to taste with salt, pepper and lemon juice. Finally, stir in the grated horseradish and bring to the boil again briefly. Serve the soup hot immediately. Decorate with the caramelised apple cubes and chopped chervil.

10.5.5 Curry lentil soup with baked cauliflower

You need:

1 L of vegetable stock, 450 g of coconut milk, three and a half red peppers, 180 g of pink lentils, three medium carrots, one onion, four teaspoons of red curry paste, half a head of cauliflower, 40 g of olive oil, 30 g of curry powder, salt, pepper, 30 g of lemon juice.

And here's how it works:

Divide the cauliflower into florets and marinate with olive oil and salt. Place in the oven on a baking tray and roast at 220°C for about 20-25 minutes. Then remove and drain on a kitchen towel. Wash the peppers and cut them into cubes. Peel carrots and also cut into small cubes. Clean onion and cut into cubes. Heat the olive oil and fry the pink lentils, the diced onion and the curry paste for about one minute. Fill up with coconut milk and vegetable stock. Cook for about 15 minutes at low heat. Stir again and again to prevent burning. After about 15 minutes cooking time add the carrot and the diced peppers. Season to taste with curry powder, salt, pepper and lemon juice. Serve the soup hot and decorate with the baked cauliflower florets.

10.5.6 Potato and mushroom soup

You need:

210 g of waxy potatoes, 260 g of mushrooms, a stick of leek (approx. 200 g), 700 g of vegetable stock, 100 g of cream, a tablespoon of rapeseed oil, salt, pepper, marjoram.

And here's how it works:

Peel the potatoes and cut into cubes. Clean and slice the mushrooms. Wash the leeks under running water until there is no sand left. Then cut into slices of about 2 cm thick. Pluck the marjoram. Fry half of the mushrooms in some rapeseed oil and season with salt and pepper. Dry them on a kitchen roll and put them aside for decoration. Heat the rapeseed oil in a pot. Add the potatoes, mushrooms and leek and sauté for about two minutes. Fill up with vegetable stock and cream and let it simmer for about 15 minutes at a mild heat. Use a blender to blend the soup to a creamy consistency. Season to taste with salt and pepper. Serve the soup very hot and decorate with the mushroom slices and plucked marjoram.

10.5.7 Chorizo stew

You need:

380 g of vine tomatoes, 200 g of chorizo, four cloves of garlic, 150 g of potatoes, one red pepper, one green pepper, one medium courgette, one bunch of soup greens, one spring onion, three tablespoons of tomato paste, one tablespoon of white wine vinegar, one bunch of fresh oregano, 750 g of vegetable stock, 30 g of rapeseed oil, salt, pepper

And here's how it works:

Cut the chorizo into strips. Clean and wash all the vegetables and cut them into cubes of about 2 cm. Heat the rapeseed oil and sauté the vegetables for about two to three minutes. Add tomato paste and after about another minute add vegetable stock. Cook for 25-30 minutes. Season to taste with salt, pepper and chilli powder and serve hot. Be careful with the salt at first, as the sausage itself is very salty. Chorizo is a spicy, firm, coarse-grained raw sausage from Spain and Portugal based on pork, seasoned with paprika and garlic.

10.5.8 French onion soup

You need:

5 large vegetable onions, 30 g of butter, 20 g of flour, 100 g of white wine, 1.4 litres of beef stock, 1 bay leaf, 4 stalks of thyme, salt, pepper, 8 slices of baguette, 70 g of grated Gruyere.

And here's how it works:

Peel onions and cut into strips. Sauté in melted butter. Add the flour and fry for one minute. Fill up with white wine and stock, add the bay leaf and simmer for about 30 minutes over a mild heat. Remove the bay leaf, add the chopped fresh thyme and simmer gently for another ten minutes. Arrange the soup in hot soup plates, cover with baguette slices and put grated cheese on the bread slices and bake at high top heat.

10.5.9 Minestrone

You need:

250 g of white beans, a bunch of vegetables, 20 g of parsley, 20 g of thyme, 20 g of bay leaf, 1 bunch of basil, 200 g of olive oil, salt, 140 g of grated Parmesan cheese, 60 g of pine nuts.

1 medium broccoli, 1 celery, 200 g of vine tomatoes, 40 g of olive oil, 20 g of tomato paste, salt, pepper, 1 small

chilli pepper, 200 g of green beans, 2 small carrots, 1 fennel bulb, 1 medium courgette.

And here's how it works:

Soak the beans overnight. The next day, rinse and cook for about two to three hours with the bundle of vegetables, some bay leaf, thyme and parsley. Do not add salt, otherwise the beans will not soften. Roast the pine nuts in a pan without fat. Mix the olive oil, parmesan, pine nuts in a mixer to make a pesto.

Clean the broccoli and cut into florets. Wash the celery and cut into strips. Clean and halve the beans. Peel and chop the carrots. Wash and chop the courgette.

Sauté the vegetables in some olive oil. Add tomato paste. Add the bean stock and cook for 35 minutes. Season to taste with salt, pepper and some garlic. Serve hot together with the pesto.

10.5.10 Lentil soup with spinach

You need:

90 g of onions, 180 g of carrots, 80 g of celeriac, a stick of leek, 80 g of dates without stones, a bunch of leaf parsley, 40 g of olive oil, 240 g of mountain lentils, 1l of chicken stock, a teaspoon of cinnamon, 200 g of baby leaf spinach, 140 g of yoghurt, 20 g of lemon juice, salt,

pepper, six styles of mint, 10 g of Ducca (North African spice mix), one salted lemon.

Salt lemons are a speciality of North African cuisine. The lemons are pickled in brine and are an ingredient of many traditional dishes. For the spice mixture Ducca, sesame and nuts are combined with coriander, cumin, mint and thyme.

And here's how it works:
Wash or clean the celery, carrots, onions and leeks and cut them into pieces about 1 cm in size. Cut dates finely. Drain and thinly slice the lemon and chop finely. Wash, dry and finely chop the parsley. Heat the oil in a large pot. Steam onions, carrots, celery, leek and 20 g of Ducca over medium heat for two to three minutes. Add lentils, salt, lemon and dates. Add the stock and 300 g of water and cook. Add the cinnamon and parsley and cook over medium heat for about 50 minutes, stirring constantly. Wash the spinach and spin dry. Puree the soup with a blender for about five seconds. Season to taste with salt and pepper, add the spinach and serve hot. Sprinkle with the yoghurt.

10.5.11 Carrot soup with spelt croutons
You need:
400 g of carrots, two medium-sized onions, 100 g of white balsamic vinegar, 30 g of ginger, 20g of olive oil, 500

g of vegetable stock, 300 g of coconut milk, salt, erythritol, ground white pepper, two medium-sized red chillies, two slices of spelt bread, 20 g of butter, half a bunch of chives.

And here's how it works:

Peel carrots, peel onions and cut into cubes. Clean the ginger and cut into fine strips. Cut carrots into cubes. Halve and roughly chop the chillies. Heat the olive oil in a medium-sized pot and fry the carrots together with the ginger, onions and chillies. Top up with the vegetable stock. Cook for about 20 minutes and then add the coconut milk and vinegar. Finish the soup with a blender. Season to taste with salt, erythritol, ground pepper and chilli.

Cut the spelt bread into cubes and lightly toast in butter. Serve the soup on plates preheated in the oven, the spelt croutons and chopped chives.

10.5.12 Parsley root soup

You need:

One kilo of parsley root, 120 g of floury potatoes, two medium sized onions, 40 g of rapeseed oil, 200 g of dry white wine, 20 g of vegetable stock (instant), one medium sized apple for example Boskoop, 200 g of whipped cream, salt, pepper, nutmeg, erythritol.

And here's how it works:

Peel and wash the parsley root and separate about 150 g of it. Cut the rest roughly. Peel, wash and chop the potatoes. Peel and chop the onions. Fry the onions together with the parsley roots in a pot with hot oil. Deglaze with white wine, a quarter litre of water and the vegetable stock, then bring to the boil. After about 20 minutes add the cream and puree. Season to taste with salt, pepper, nutmeg and erythritol. Fry the remaining parsley roots with the finely diced potatoes in a pan, sprinkle with some erythritol. Serve the soup on plates preheated in the oven and garnish with the caramelized potato and apple cubes.

10.5.13 Turnips Potato soup with wild garlic Pesto

You need:

One medium onion, 20 g of rapeseed oil, 400 g of rutabaga, 350 g of potatoes, floury cooking, 20 g of vegetable stock (instant), 20 g of red curry paste, 50 g of cream, 80 g of pine nuts, 60 g of wild garlic, 40 g of olive oil, 40 g of sliced Parmesan cheese, salt, pepper, erythritol.

And here's how it works:

Wash the turnips and cut into large cubes. Do the same with the potatoes. Peel and dice the onions. Heat the rapeseed oil in a medium-sized pot and sauté the turnips together with the potatoes. Deglaze with 700 g of water and the vegetable stock. Add the cream and the curry paste. Use a blender to make a homogeneous soup. Lightly roast the pine nuts without fat in a pan - let them cool down. Puree into a pesto together with the olive oil, wild garlic, parmesan, salt, pepper and some erythritol. Serve the soup on plates preheated in the oven and garnish with pine-bear-garlic pesto.

Wild garlic is a relative of garlic, onion and chives. It has white flowers and was already known to the Romans and Germanic tribes as a spice and medicinal plant. Bear's garlic contains vitamin C, essential oils, magnesium and iron. Although it tastes similar to garlic, it does not affect mouth and body odour.

10.5.14 Lentil soup with chard and minced meat
You need:

Two medium sized peppers, a lemon, 70 g of chard, 260 g of pink lentils, 150 g of minced beef, 20 g of caraway seeds, 10 g of cumin, 20 g of butter, 25 g of vegetable stock (instant), 10 g of ginger, a clove of garlic, a medium sized onion.

And here's how it works:

Wash the chard, then cut into 3 cm pieces. Halve the pepperoni and process into fine slices. Clean and chop the garlic clove. Remove ginger from the skin and cut into cubes. Heat the butter in a medium-sized pot and fry the onions, garlic, ginger, cumin and caraway seeds for about

20 seconds. Add minced beef and fry gently. Add lentils, pour water and vegetable broth. Cook over a mild heat for about 20 minutes until the mixture is creamy. Add the chard five minutes before the end of the cooking time. Season to taste with lemon juice, salt and pepper. Serve the soup on plates preheated in the oven and garnish with the peppers.

10.5.15 Kohlrabi Savoy Soup

You need:

200 g of kohlrabi, 200 g of savoy cabbage, one medium onion, one medium potato, 20 g of butter, 100 g of white wine, 20 g of vegetable stock (instant), 100 g of cream cheese, salt, pepper, nutmeg, half bunch of chervil.

And here's how it works:

Wash, clean and dice the kohlrabi, savoy cabbage and potatoes. Peel and chop the onion. Heat the butter in a medium-sized pot and sauté the kohlrabi, savoy cabbage, onions and potatoes in it. After two minutes, drain with 750 g water and the white wine and vegetable stock. Season the cream cheese with salt, pepper and nutmeg and shape into cams using a teaspoon.

Serve the soup on plates preheated in the oven and garnish with the cream cheese curls and sliced chervil.

10.5.16 Spicy noodle soup with chicken

You need:

Coriander seed, one chilli pepper, dried, ¼ bunch of mint, salt, pepper, 1 onion, one green pepper green, 320 g of chicken breast fillet, 50 g of olive oil, 200g of vermicelli, 2 tablespoons of erythritol, 350 g of tomatoes peeled, two bay leaves, 1 tsp paprika powder, 1 tbsp of cumin seed, 1 tbsp of oregano, ½ tsp of pigment ground, 1.3 L of poultry stock, one red onion, one bunch of coriander green, one firm avocado, juice of half a lime

And here's how it works:

Roast dried chilli, cumin and coriander seeds in a pan without fat. Mix everything together with salt small mortars. Dice onion and garlic. Cut pepper without seeds into strips. Cut the chicken meat into cubes of approx. 3 cm and season.

Sauté the meat in hot olive oil. Add onions and garlic and fry until transparent. Add remaining spices and tomatoes to the meat. Steam for about four minutes until the tomatoes burst open. Add the pasta and chicken stock and cook for about 20 minutes.

Cut red onions into rings. Chop the coriander. Pluck mint. Clean the avocado and cut the flesh into pieces of about 3 cm. Mix the soup with salt, pepper, coriander green, mint, avocado cubes and onions and arrange on plates preheated in the oven.

10.6 Salad dressings

Most salad dressings in supermarket refrigerated cabinets contain a variety of ingredients, including additives and preservatives. These ingredients are unhealthy, expensive and superfluous. Making salad dressings yourself is healthier and requires little effort.

10.6.1 Vinaigrette, classic
You need:
For the classic of all salad sauces you need one part vinegar, lemon juice or another acid and three parts oil. The oil can be based on sunflowers, rape, sesame, olives, etc. It is important that the oil is the first pressing. For frying and cooking we prefer high quality olive oil from the first pressing. If a taste-intensive vinegar, for example old white wine vinegar, is used, a tasteless oil should be used and vice versa.

A typical basic recipe is: 100 g of white wine vinegar, 400 g of rape seed oil, half a tablespoon of mustard, a tablespoon of erythritol, salt, pepper, half a teaspoon of garlic.

And here's how it works:
The most common mistake made when making a vinaigrette: all the ingredients are mixed together in a container with a hand blender. This procedure causes the

oil to settle and the salad dressing to taste oily. The principle is as follows: an emulsifier is needed, for example mustard or egg yolk. First you put a tablespoon of mustard, salt, erythritol or honey, pepper, a little garlic and the white wine vinegar in the container. In the second course, the oil is mixed in, first drop by drop, then in larger quantities. The result will be a homogeneous, round tasting salad dressing where the oil will not settle permanently. If you are looking for a special variant, white wine vinegar is replaced by e.g. raspberry vinegar and the addition of fresh raspberries.

10.6.2 Yoghurt dressing

You need:

For the basic version of a yoghurt dressing: 300 g of yoghurt, 50 g of white wine vinegar, 40 g of rapeseed oil, two teaspoons of mustard, salt, pepper and erythritol or honey.

And here's how it works:

Mix all the ingredients in a bowl and with a whisk—done. If you want to make the sauce spicier, use garlic and chilli. Another variation is to add freshly cut chives and pink pepper berries to the base. If you prefer Asian flavours, use ginger, freshly cut coriander and cayenne pepper.

10.6.3 Wasabi lime dressing

You need:

100 g of sour cream, 110 g of olive oil, 200 g of apple juice, one tablespoon of wasabi paste, one lime, a small piece of ginger root, salt, pepper, erythritol.

And here's how it works:

Clean and finely grate the ginger, wash the lime warm and grate the peel. Halve the lime and squeeze it. Mix ginger, lime zest, lime juice, wasabi, sour cream, apple juice in a bowl. Add olive oil slowly and then quickly. Season to taste with salt, pepper, erythritol. This salad dressing reminds of a horseradish dressing. It goes very well with, for example, a lamb's lettuce with croutons and bacon.

Wasabi is green, hot, comes from the land of smiles and is also called Japanese horseradish. For a long time it was known exclusively to friends of Asian cuisine. Mixed with soy sauce, it is a must for every sushi dish.

10.6.4 Buttermilk-blackberry dressing

You need:

100 g of lettuce, 100 g of buttermilk, 150 g of crème fraîche, two tablespoons of balsamic vinegar, two tablespoons of maple syrup, 50 g of fresh blackberries, salt, pepper, erythritol.

And here's how it works:

Hold back half of the blackberries. Puree the other ingredients in a bowl using a hand blender. Cut the remaining blackberries into quarters and stir into the dressing. Pureed lettuce will bind the blackberries at this point. Alternatively, iceberg, lamb's lettuce or lollo rosso could be used.

10.6.5 Cranberry and hazelnut dressing

You need:

50 g of erythritol, 50 g of cranberry, four tablespoons of water, 20 g of medium hot mustard, 50 g of white wine vinegar, 50 g of hazelnut oil, 150 g of rapeseed oil.

And here's how it works:

Caramelise erythritol in a small pot until brown. Add cranberries and water, cover and simmer gently for about five minutes until the caramel has dissolved. Then let the cranberries cool down and puree them with a hand blender. Mix mustard, cranberries, vinegar, salt, erythritol and pepper. Slowly stir the hazelnut oil and rapeseed oil into the mixture.

Cranberries, also called cranberries, are sweet and sour tasting berries originally from North America. They have a high content of secondary plant substances and thus have a positive effect on the intestinal flora and against urinary tract infections. Their taste is reminiscent of cranberries and they are often served as compote with game dishes at Christmas time.

10.6.6 Pea and balm dressing

You need:

100 g of frozen peas, a bunch of lemon balm, 20 g of white wine, 100 g of vegetable stock, 200 g of rapeseed oil, salt, pepper, erythritol.

And here's how it works:

Blanch deep-frozen peas in lightly salted water for about three minutes. Leave to cool. Mix the peas, lemon balm, white wine, salt, pepper, erythritol, garlic in a container, then stir in the vegetable stock and finally the rapeseed oil using a hand blender.

This salad dressing is perfect with rustic pasta salads, for example, an Italian pasta salad with olives, cucumber, bresaola and shaved parmesan. Lemon balm is a must for any balcony or garden planting. It belongs to the classic kitchen and medicinal herbs. Its lemon fragrance makes it a popular and versatile component of traditional dishes. Its ingredients help against restlessness and stomach problems.

10.6.7 Mango-Jalapeño Dressing

You need:

One large mango, two fresh red jalapeños, a clove of garlic, a lime, 40 g of olive oil, a large red onion, 100 g of orange juice, 20 g of liquid honey, salt, pepper.

And here's how it works:

Cut the mango in half, remove the core, remove the mango flesh and dice coarsely. Peel the garlic clove and cut into pieces. Grate the lime peel and extract the juice. Peel the red onion and cut into fine cubes. Wash the jalapeños, cut them in half, remove the seeds and cut into rings. Fry the mango cubes and finely chopped jalapeños in a little olive oil, add the honey. Add the juice of orange and lime as well as their rubbing. Leave to cool, then puree. Stir in olive oil and finally add red onion and the rest of the jalapeños.

Excellent with a colourful leaf salad with fried chicken breast and baguette bread. Jalapeño is one of the most popular chilli varieties. They are characterised by a strong but tolerable pungency. The vitamin-rich Mexican pod is often used in salsas, baked or pickled in vinegar.

10.6.8 Blueberry pumpernickel dressing

You need:

110 g of pumpernickel, 140 g of blueberries, 120 g of blueberry juice, 30 g of apple vinegar, 60 g of olive oil, one orange, salt, pepper, one tablespoon of blueberry jam.

And here's how it works:

Set half of the blueberries aside. Cut the pumpernickel into small pieces. Grate the orange peel. Juice the orange.

Mix all ingredients in a tall container with a hand blender to a homogenous mass.

This dressing is particularly suitable in winter as a salad dressing or marinade. Pumpernickel is a speciality from Westphalia and consists of rye meal, salt and water. Pumpernickel is baked for about 24 hours and therefore caramelised. This gives the bread its own sweet note.

10.7 Smoothie

Smoothies usually have a high nutrient density and may be full of carbohydrates in the form of fructose. You should therefore not drink these drinks regularly and in large quantities. If you need to mix for more than 90 seconds, add ice cubes or cold water to prevent the drinks from heating up and losing their ingredients. Fibrous leaf green is often used in the recipes. If your blender reaches its limits, you can replace the ingredients with baby spinach, lamb's lettuce or lettuce, for example. Another disadvantage of smoothies: they offer nothing to chew and are therefore detrimental to dental health.

Green smoothies are mainly vegetable-based and are full of vitamins, secondary plant compounds, minerals and amino acids and are therefore preferable to fruit smoothies.

10.7.1 Chinese Cabbage Blueberry Smoothie
You need:
80 g of blueberries, one orange, one banana, 100 g of water, four medium sized leaves of Chinese cabbage
And here's how it works:
Remove the peel from the orange and banana and puree all ingredients with a high-speed mixer until creamy. Blueberries contain a lot of water and are low in calories. They contain a high proportion of provitamin A and

vitamin C, which is said to prevent cell damage. Main ingredients of China Cabbage:

In addition to anthocyanins, vitamins and minerals, special tanning agents also make blueberries healthy. Tanning agents act against diarrhoea, inhibit the reproduction of bacteria and accelerate the healing of mucous membrane inflammations. This effect is, however, mainly observed with dried blueberries.

10.7.2 Green Detox Smoothie

You need:

140 g of kale, a piece of apple, half a banana, a cucumber, juice and peel of half a lemon, 240 g of water, a teaspoon of wheatgrass powder.

And here's how it works:

Wash the kale thoroughly. Then spin dry using a salad spinner. Do not peel the cucumber, just clean it in water with a vegetable brush. Cut it in half lengthwise and remove the seeds. Do not peel the apple, just remove the core. Cut the apple into small pieces. Mix all ingredients in a high-speed mixer to a creamy drink.

Wheatgrass powder belongs to the Super Foods and is said to strengthen the immune system and have a positive effect on the eyesight.

Kale stimulates digestion and helps us lose weight. It contains valuable fibre, which is important for our intestines and for good digestion. In addition, kale keeps us full longer due to the fibre and prevents ravenous appetite attacks, as it keeps the blood sugar level constant.

10.7.3 Sauerkraut-Grapefruit Smoothie

You need:

Half a grapefruit, 100 g of sauerkraut, half a pear, half an apple, a teaspoon of nut oil

And here's how it works:

Halve the grapefruit and remove the skin. Blend all ingredients together with 100 g of water and a hand blender.

Sauerkraut with its lactic acid bacteria will make your digestion work. The pectin contained in the peel of pear and apple activates the bladder and kidney function. The grapefruit masks the taste of the sauerkraut. The nut oil contributes to the taste and ensures that fat-soluble vitamins can be absorbed by the body. Grapefruit contains minerals such as potassium, calcium, magnesium, iron and phosphate. The plant substance naringin is responsible for the bitter taste of the fruit.

10.7.4 Avocado-Banana-Apple Smoothie

You need:

A handful of spinach, a Boskoop apple, a medium-sized banana, the flesh of a quarter avocado, the juice of an orange, 20 g of ginger, 200 g of water.

And here's how it works:

Wash and clean all components. Do not peel the apple, just remove the core. Blend all ingredients in a high-speed mixer to a creamy drink. If necessary, increase the amount of water. Avocados are rich in unsaturated fatty acids and have a fat content of up to 30%. They are rich in minerals, especially magnesium, potassium and iron.

10.7.5 Chick peas smoothie, Greek yoghurt and broccoli

You need:

140 g of Greek yoghurt, a tablespoon of almonds, 70 g of broccoli, 70 g of strawberries, 30 g of chickpeas, 180 g of cold green tea, a quarter teaspoon of cinnamon.

And here's how it works:

Roast the almonds briefly in a pan without fat. Wash the strawberries and remove the green. Wash and dry the broccoli. Blend all ingredients together in a fast rotating mixer until creamy. Green tea contains plenty of caffeine and provides the necessary boost when consumed in the morning. Good for slimming.

Broccoli contains a high dose of vital substances. These include vitamin B complexes as well as vitamins C, E and K, the minerals calcium, magnesium, iron, zinc and potassium and a large number of secondary plant substances that have a strong antioxidant effect.

10.7.6 Spinach and savoy cabbage smoothie with pear

You need:
80 g of fresh savoy cabbage, 80 g of baby spinach, two untreated pears, an apple, if possible Boskoop, half a bunch of mint, one tablespoon of honey.

And here's how it works:
Clean the savoy cabbage and apples, remove the core. Wash and chop the savoy cabbage. Clean the baby spinach. Puree all ingredients together with 400 g of water in a suitable container using a hand blender.

Savoy cabbage contains glucosinolates. These sulphur-containing molecules give it its strong, spicy aroma and protect the cabbage from predators in nature. In the human body they can have an antioxidant effect.

10.7.7 Ginger Grape Carrot Smoothie
You need:

240 g of carrots, 90 g of seedless red grapes, 20 g of fresh ginger, one tablespoon of rapeseed oil, 50 g of mineral water.

And here's how it works:

Remove the green at the end of the carrots. Brush under water, grate roughly with the skin. Clean the ginger. Blend all the other ingredients in a blender or hand blender. The oil once again ensures that the fat-soluble vitamins are absorbed by the body. Ginger has an anti-inflammatory effect. Red grapes have a high content of B vitamins.

Ginger contains essential oils and gingerol, which gives it its pungency. In addition, the small tuber contains digestive and circulation stimulating substances such as Borneol and Cineol. Vitamin C, iron, magnesium, calcium, potassium, phosphorus and sodium are also contained. Ginger is therefore not only a tasty food, but also a remedy.

10.7.8 Pineapple-Mango Detox Smoothie

You need:

An orange, 180 g of coconut water, half a mango, ¼ pineapple, juice and peel of half a lime, some cayenne pepper.

And here's how it works:

Remove the peel from the orange. Cut the mango in half, remove the core and remove the flesh. Cut the pineapple into quarters and remove the flesh from the skin and stalk. Blend all ingredients together with a hand blender. Add a pinch of salt to add flavour. Season to taste with a little cayenne pepper.

Just like tomatoes, watermelons, carrots or oranges, pineapple has a diuretic effect. This is due to potassium—it drains. The fibre and the enzyme bromelain help the intestines to get rid of toxins better. It also contains vitamin C.

10.8 Healthy breakfast

10.8.1 Skyr with seeds, oranges and banana
You need:
10 g of coconut chips, 15 g of cashew nuts, 15 g of walnut kernels, 15 g of almond kernels, 15 g of pine nuts, one banana, two oranges, 600 g of skyr, 10 g of puffed amaranth.

And here's how it works:
Roast the seeds and coconut chips in a pan without fat and let them cool down. Mix the juice and grated orange with the Skyr. Remove the remaining orange peel and cut into slices. Spread the Skyr on peels and sprinkle the roasted seeds on top. Decorate with amaranth.

Skyr is a speciality from Iceland, which is low in fat and at the same time rich in protein and reminiscent of low-fat curd cheese. Amaranth can be called a pseudo-cereal, as it is a grass species. It is extremely healthy and produces grains that contain starch but are gluten-free.

10.8.2 Spelt bread with avocado cream and graved salmon
You need:
Two fully ripe avocados, juice of half a lemon, 180 g of cream cheese, a bunch of spring onions, 10 g of chopped parsley, salt, colourful pepper from the mill, three

radishes, ⅓ Cucumber, 30 g of sprouts—for example radish sprouts, a box of cress, four slices of wholemeal spelt bread, 200 g of gravlax.

And here's how it works:

Wash and slice the spring onions, cut the avocado in half, remove the core, remove the flesh, mash finely with a fork. Sprinkle the avocado with the juice of the lemon so that it does not discolour. Wash, clean and slice the radish and cucumber. Mix the cream cheese with the avocado and add the parsley. Season to taste with salt, pepper and the rest of the lemon. Toast wholemeal bread. Spread the avocado cream on top and cover with slices of radish and cucumber. Place the salmon on top and garnish with radish sprouts and cress.

Avocado is also called butter of the forest because of its high fat content. This fruit has a high content of unsaturated fatty acids, which can be easily converted into energy by your body. While avocado also has a low fructose content.

10.8.3 Birch muesli with carrot boscoop salad

You need:

25 g of grated coconut, 15 g of cashew nuts, 10 g of cranberries, 10 g of sultanas, 70 g of oatmeal, 280 g of yoghurt, 20 g of honey, a medium sized Boskoop apple, a

carrot, juice and grated lime, a pinch of erythritol, a pinch of salt.

And here's how it works:

Fry the cashew nuts and grated coconut in a pan without fat until golden brown. Wash the carrot and brush it under water. Wash and quarter the boscoop and remove the core. Leave the skin on the apple and carrot. Cut the apple and carrot into fine strips or grate them with a suitable slicer. Marinate with erythritol and salt, work through slightly and season to taste with the juice and grated lime. Mix the yoghurt, honey, oatmeal, cranberries and sultanas, leave to stand for five minutes and fill into bowls. Decorate with carrot Boskoop salad. The Boskoop is a winter apple with a particularly high acid content. Those who appreciate sour apples can enjoy this apple variety fresh as table fruit. In addition, Boskoop apples have particularly few allergens, which is why they are edible for some apple allergy sufferers.

10.8.4 Oatmeal with maple syrup and banana

You need:

60 g of oat flakes, 250 g of oat milk, 40 g of maple syrup, half a teaspoon of cinnamon, one banana, 20 g of walnuts or pine nuts, 10 g of oat flakes, 10 g of icing sugar.

And here's how it works:

Bring oat milk to boiling point in a pot, add oat flakes, stir well and leave to swell for five minutes. Add maple syrup and cinnamon. Make sure that nothing burns. Roast the walnuts or pine nuts and the oats in a pan without fat. Caramelise with icing sugar. Spread the oatmeal porridge on peels and decorate with sliced banana and the roasted seeds.

In contrast to conventional sugar, maple syrup contains some valuable minerals such as calcium, potassium, magnesium and iron. However, the energy content is only slightly below that of sugar and honey.

10.9 Mediterranean

10.9.1 Grilled Bread

You need:

500g of flour, salt, a cube of yeast, 3 tablespoons of olive oil, half a red onion, a bunch of parsley leaves, 160 ml of strained tomatoes, 20 g of pine nuts, half an organic lemon, pepper, a finely chopped clove of garlic.

And here's how it works:

Mix the flour, salt, yeast, 160 ml of warm water and a tablespoon of olive oil and work into a homogenous dough. Peel onion and cut into fine cubes. Wash parsley, dry with kitchen paper and chop finely with a sharp knife. Mix the tomato sauce, onions, parsley, pine nuts, lemon juice and grated parsley and season to taste with salt, pepper and garlic. Roll out the dough on a work surface to a height of approx. 3 cm and cut into three equally long strips. Weave the plait and spread the tomato sauce on top. Leave to rise in a warm place for another 20 minutes. Preheat the oven to 180°C and bake the Mediterranean barbecue plait for about 25 minutes.

10.9.2 Fried fillet of gilthead

You need:

750 g of triplets, salt, pepper, 30 g of chopped garlic, ½ bunch of leaf parsley, 20 g of small capers, 230 g of cherry tomatoes, 1 bunch of rocket, 60 g of olive oil, 30 g of

white wine vinegar, 20 g of liquid honey, four gilthead fillets, 20 g of butter, ½ lemon.

And here's how it works:

Wash and halve the potatoes. Then cook in salted water for about eight minutes until al dente. Peel garlic and chop finely. Wash the parsley, dry it on a kitchen roll and chop finely. Drain the capers. Wash the tomatoes, remove the greens and cut them in half, wash the arugula, dry it and chop it finely. Heat oil in a pan and fry the potatoes in it. After about four minutes, add the tomatoes, vinegar, honey, garlic, parsley and capers and cook for another two minutes. Season to taste with salt and pepper. Rinse fish fillets cold and dry them on a kitchen roll. Season with salt and pepper. Heat olive oil in a frying pan. Fry the fillets of gilthead on the skin side for about three minutes until crispy. Turn the fish fillets just before they are cooked, add the butter and fry over a low heat for another two minutes. Drizzle with lemon juice. Arrange the hot tomato potatoes on a plate. Place the fish fillet on top.

Triplets, also called small grading or field ware, are potatoes of a special size grading, regardless of the potato variety.

10.9.3 Antipasti with vegetables, mushrooms and olives

You need:

One aubergine, one courgette, one green pepper, one yellow pepper, one red pepper, 200 g of brown mushrooms, a bunch of leaf parsley, 150 g of pitted green olives, 200 g of olive oil, four cloves of garlic. Salt, pepper, 150 g of erythritol, 150 g of dark balsamic vinegar.

And here's how it works:

Wash and clean all the vegetables and cut them into strips about 2 cm wide. Do not wash the mushrooms, but brush them. Wash the leaf parsley, dab dry and chop coarsely. Clean the garlic and mix it with the salt to a garlic paste. The following procedure is an example of how this is done with courgettes. Heat olive oil in a pan. Sauté the courgette. Season with salt, pepper and garlic paste. Deglaze with 4 cl of Aceto Balsamico, add two tablespoons of Erythritol. Simmer for another 20 seconds, then remove and leave to cool in the marinade. Do the same with the rest of the vegetables. Leave to cool overnight and add salt and pepper the next day to taste. Arrange everything together with the olives on a starter plate.

10.9.4 Penne in tuna tomato sauce

You need:

500 g panicles of tomatoes, a clove of garlic, half a bunch of spring onions, a small medium hot red chilli pepper, half a pot of basil, 120 g of tuna in oil, salt, pepper, 50 g of olive oil, two shallots, 200 g of penne pasta.

And here's how it works:

Clean the garlic and dice finely. Clean and dice the shallots. Do the same with the spring onion. Clean the chillies and dice them finely. Wash the tomatoes, remove the greenery and cut into fine cubes. Heat the olive oil, sauté the shallots and garlic briefly. Add spring onion and diced tomatoes. Season with salt, pepper and basil. Simmer over a mild heat for about 30 minutes. Drain the tuna and add to the tomato sauce. Cook penne pasta according to instructions. Arrange everything together on preheated plates.

10.9.5 Pasta salad with mozzarella

You need:

400 g of spiral noodles, 200 g of tomatoes, 100g of rocket, 125g of buffalo mozzarella, half a bunch of chives, 60 g of curd cheese, 140 g of yoghurt, two tablespoons of olive oil, two tablespoons of white wine vinegar, pepper, salt, a clove of garlic.

And here's how it works:

Clean and chop the garlic. Clean and chop the chives finely. Cut mozzarella into large pieces. Cut tomatoes in half and mix with salt, erythritol, pepper and olive oil. Mix curd cheese, yoghurt, olive oil, vinegar, salt and pepper to a salad dressing. Cook the spiral noodles in plenty of salted water, rinse cold. Mix with cherry tomatoes, rocket and mozzarella and garnish with chives.

10.9.6 Braised meatballs

You need:

280 g of green beans, 490 g of small potatoes, 60 g of pine nuts, 100 g of tomatoes, half a bunch of thyme, 460 g of mixed mince, 45 g of breadcrumbs, one egg, salt, pepper, one red and yellow pepper, one medium red onion, 60 g of olive oil, 60 g of tomato paste, 1 teaspoon of vegetable stock (instant).

And here's how it works:

Wash and peel the potatoes and cook them in lightly salted water for about five minutes until al dente. In the meantime, clean and wash the beans. Add the beans to the potatoes and cook for another eight minutes. Roast the pine nuts in a hot pan without fat. Wash the tomatoes, remove the greens and cut them into small pieces. Clean the thyme and chop finely. Chop the pine nuts. Mix the minced meat, breadcrumbs, egg, thyme, pine nuts and tomatoes. Season with salt and pepper. Form about six meatballs from the resulting mixture. Wash and clean the peppers, remove the core and cut into pieces. Peel onions and cut into strips. Fry the meatballs in hot fat for about three minutes on each side, remove and put aside. Lightly fry the bell peppers and the onions. Add tomato paste and cook for another two minutes. Deglaze with ¼ litres of water. Add stock, potatoes and beans and braise for another four minutes. Add the meatballs and cook for about six minutes until done.

10.10 Vegan dishes

10.10.1 Baked aubergine and carrots

You need:

200 g of celeriac, 2 tablespoons of rapeseed oil, salt, a medium sized aubergine, 40 g of soy sauce, six carrots with green, oil for frying, 50 g starch, pepper, erythritol, 1 tablespoon of light balsamic vinegar, 1 tablespoon of agave syrup, 1 vanilla pod, a small red medium hot chilli pod.

And here's how it works:

Wash, clean and dice the celery. Lightly fry the cubes in 20 g of rapeseed oil, drain with a little water and season with a pinch of salt. Cover with a lid and cook until soft. Wash the aubergine, cut it into slices about 2 cm thick and marinate with the soy sauce.

Brush the carrots, slightly shorten the green and clean the carrot. Turn aubergine slices in the starch. Heat one litre of fat to fry the aubergine in it. Halve the vanilla pod and remove the pulp. Cut the chilli pepper into small cubes.

Puree the celery with a blender and season with light balsamic vinegar, salt, erythritol and pepper. Heat the agave syrup and cook the carrots together with the diced chillies, vanilla pod and pulp in it.

10.10.2 Pak Choi with ginger-garlic sauce and sesame

You need:

750 g of pak choi, two bunches of spring onions, 20 g of ginger, two cloves of garlic, three dried chillies, 40 g of rapeseed oil, 15 g of erythritol, salt, pepper, 30 g of soy sauce, 20 g of dark balsamic vinegar, 5 g of cornflour, 50 g of white sesame, 300 g of brown rice, 200 g of vegetable stock.

And here's how it works:

Clean and finely chop the spring onions, ginger, garlic and chillies. Heat 20 g of rapeseed oil in a pan and lightly sauté the previously cut vegetables for two minutes. Then top up with soy sauce, vinegar and 150 g of water. Mix cornflour with 30 g of water to thicken the above sauce. Lightly roast sesame seeds in a pan without fat. Clean and wash Pak Choi and divide into individual leaves. Cook the rice in slightly salted water. Sauté Pak Choi in 20 g of rapeseed oil until colourless, deglaze with vegetable broth and steam for three minutes, covered. Arrange the Pak Choi vegetables on a plate preheated in the oven, pour the sauce over them and decorate with sesame seeds. Serve with brown brown rice.

Pak Choi has season from June to September. It strengthens the immune system, protects the body cells, is good for pregnant women. In Europe it is also called Chinese mustard cabbage or Chinese leafy cabbage.

10.10.3 Tomatoes stuffed with oriental couscous

You need:

200 g of couscous, 60 g of sultanas, salt, pepper, 55 g of pine nuts, 1.5 tsp of coriander seeds, ½ pot of mint, 200 g of large beef tomatoes, 2 tbsp of olive oil, 1 tbsp of hot curry powder, 20 g of rapeseed oil.

And here's how it works:

Roast the pine nuts in a pan without fat. Pour double the amount of hot water over the couscous and sultanas and leave to stand. Coarsely crush the coriander seeds in a mortar. Wash, dry and finely chop the mint. Wash the tomatoes, remove the green and cut in half. Remove the inside of the tomatoes and dice. Clean the garlic and chop finely. Mix the couscous with mint, coriander seeds, salt, pepper, finely chopped tomato cubes, garlic and the curry powder and fill into the tomato halves. Bake at 180 degrees in a preheated oven for about 30 minutes.

10.10.4 Bami Goreng with broccoli and tempeh

You need:

220 g of Mie noodles, 280 g of Tempeh, 140 g of pink mushrooms, 220 g of young wild broccoli, a bunch of spring onions, 40 g of rapeseed oil, 20 g of light soy sauce, 100 g of vegetable stock, 10 g of Sambal Olek, 30 g of

roasted sesame seeds. For the marinade: a clove of garlic, 20 g of light soy sauce, 20 g of dark soy sauce, 10 g of maple syrup, 10 g of sesame oil

And here's how it works:

Finely grate the clove of garlic and mix the remaining ingredients for the marinade. Cut the tempeh into 5 × 5 cm pieces and leave to stand in the garlic marinade for at least an hour. Cook the pasta in lightly salted water, drain and rinse cold. Sauté the tempeh and remaining vegetables in rapeseed oil until colourless, then deglaze with the vegetable stock, soy sauce and sambal olek. Add the noodles, stir and season to taste with salt. Serve on plates preheated in the oven and decorate with the roasted sesame seeds.

Tempeh is an important source of protein and comes from Asia. Like tofu, it is made from soybeans. Tempeh is inoculated with a noble mould and then fermented and stored for two days. This gives the product a slightly nutty taste. Available in the trade as a pressed bar product.

10.10.5 Sweet potato, chickpeas and almond sauce

You need:

450 g of pre-cooked chickpeas, 10g of ground cumin, 5g of ground cinnamon, 5g of ground coriander, 5 g of paprika powder, salt, pepper, 20 g of lime juice, 50 g of almond milk, erythritol, half a bunch of chervil, 220 g of

cherry tomatoes, 20 g of olive oil, 850 g of sweet potatoes, two cloves of garlic, 50 g of sesame paste.

And here's how it works:

Peel sweet potatoes, cut into 2 cm thick oblong slices, cut cherry tomatoes in half. Make a sauce from almond milk, lime juice, garlic and the sesame paste and put aside. Mix the sweet potatoes and chickpeas with all the other ingredients. Preheat the oven to 180°C. Line a baking tray with baking paper. Put marinated sweet potato and chick peas on the baking tray and cook for 50 minutes. After half the cooking time add the cherry tomatoes. Arrange the sweet potato and chickpea tomato mix on plates, decorate with the sauce and chopped chervil.

10.10.6 Courgette spaghetti with lentil bolognese

You need:

Three large courgettes, two large onions, 50 g of garlic, 150 g of carrots, 50 g of olive oil, 350 g of pink lentils, 800 g of tomatoes, 30 g of tomato paste, 10 g oregano, salt, pepper.

And here's how it works:

Cut the courgette into noodles with a spiral cutter. Wash and peel the carrots and cut them into fine cubes. Do the same with onions, garlic and tomatoes. Lightly fry the sliced vegetables in olive oil and add tomatoes and tomato paste. Simmer for two minutes. Then add the pink lentils and pour in the vegetable stock. Cook covered for 15 minutes. Add oregano. Season to taste with salt and pepper. Heat olive oil in a frying pan, add the courgette pasta, season with salt and cook covered for three minutes.

10.10.7 Baked aubergine, celery puree, carrots

You need:

200 g of celeriac, 2 tablespoons of rapeseed oil, salt, one medium sized aubergine, 40 g of soy sauce, six carrots with green, oil for frying, 50 g of starch, pepper, erythritol, 1 tablespoon of light balsamic vinegar, 1 tablespoon of agave syrup, one vanilla pod, one small red medium hot chilli pod.

And here's how it works:

Wash, clean and dice the celery. Lightly fry the cubes in 20 g of rapeseed oil, add a little water and season with a pinch of salt. Cover with a lid and cook until soft. Wash the aubergine, cut it into slices about 2 cm thick and marinate with the soy sauce.

Brush the carrots, slightly shorten the green and clean the carrot. Turn aubergine slices in the starch. Heat one litre of fat to fry the aubergine in it. Halve the vanilla pod and remove the pulp. Cut the chilli pepper into small cubes.

Puree the celery with a blender and season with light balsamic vinegar, salt, erythritol and pepper. Heat the agave syrup and cook the carrots together with the diced chillies, vanilla pod and pulp in it.

10.11 Snacks

10.11.1 Leek-Paprika Muffin

You need:

Two spring onions, one red pepper, one clove of garlic, two tablespoons of olive oil, half a bunch of basil, one egg, 50 ml of milk, 150 g of low-fat curd, salt, pepper, 40 g of grated Emmental cheese, 190 g of wholemeal spelt flour, a sachet of baking powder, a teaspoon of baking soda.

And here's how it works:

Clean the spring onion, peppers and garlic and cut into cubes of about 2 cm. Heat the olive oil and steam the vegetables for about five minutes. Season with salt and pepper. In a bowl mix quark, milk, egg, Emmental, spelt flour, baking powder and baking soda. Spread the mixture evenly in muffin cups and bake in a preheated oven at 180°C for about 30 minutes. Muffins can be combined with vegetable dips or a crisp salad.

Leeks are one of the few foods with a high inulin content. Inulin is a soluble fibre with extremely beneficial effects on the intestinal flora, which is why inulin is often taken as a food supplement as part of a healthy intestinal flora build-up.

10.11.2 Arancini - Sicilian rice balls

You need:

120 g of risotto rice, 60 g of frozen peas, salt, pepper, 40 g of flour, 60 g of breadcrumbs, one egg, 45 g of cooked ham, 20 g of olive oil, 500 ml of vegetable stock, 7 g of grated Parmesan cheese, two shallots, 500 ml of rapeseed oil.

And here's how it works:

Finely dice the cooked ham. Defrost the peas. Clean the shallots and cut into cubes. Heat olive oil, sauté shallots in it, add risotto rice. Cook the rice while stirring constantly. Add grated parmesan. Let the mixture cool down. Add flour, peas and boiled ham to the risotto mixture and mix. Form evenly sized balls. Heat rapeseed oil. Turn the rice balls in the breadcrumbs and bake in hot rapeseed oil. Drain them on kitchen paper and let them cool down.

Arancini are fried and stuffed rice balls. They are part of the traditional Sicilian cuisine and, depending on the province, are conical in shape or filled with cheese or other vegetables.

10.11.3 Spinach Crostini au gratin

You need:

150 g cream cheese, a medium shallot, 100 g of grated mountain cheese, 30g of pine nuts, salt, pepper, 20 g of

olive oil, two cloves of garlic, 110 g of leaf spinach, 300 g of ciabatta bread.

And here's how it works:

Sort and wash the spinach. Roast the pine nuts in a pan without fat. Clean and chop the shallot. Heat olive oil and sauté the diced shallots. Add cream cheese and spinach. Heat up for two minutes. Finally add the mountain cheese. Stir until the mountain cheese has melted. Let the mixture cool down. Cut the ciabatta bread into 2 cm thick slices and fry in a pan with olive oil. Spread the spinach mixture evenly on top and gratinate over the top when the heat is high.

Spinach contains a lot of vitamin C. This reduces the effect of the oxalic acid contained in green vegetables.

10.12 Sweet reward

10.12.1 Coffee Cream
You need:
300 g milk, five sheets of white gelatine, three egg yolks, 30 g of erythritol, 200 g of whipped cream, eight amarettini, cocoa powder, one vanilla pod.

And here's how it works:
Soak the gelatine in cold water. Halve the vanilla pod and scrape out the pulp. Bring the pulp and pod to the boil with 250 g of milk and allow it to stand for a few minutes. Mix the egg yolks together with the erythritol in a bowl. Bring the milk briefly to the boil again and stir into the egg mixture. Stir constantly with a whisk. Squeeze the gelatine and add it to the hot mixture. Add the coffee powder. Chill the mixture and stir occasionally. Whip the cream until stiff. Just before the coffee cream starts to gel, carefully fold in the whipped cream. Then pour the mixture into four coffee cups and leave to cool for at least four hours. Coarsely crumble the Amarettini. Process the remaining milk into milk foam. Decorate the coffee cream with the milk foam and the crumbled Amarettini.

10.12.2 Ricotta cheesecake - hazelnut caramel
You need:
700 g of ricotta, 110 g of maple syrup, one vanilla pod, 190 g of flour, 70 g of erythritol, 125 g of butter, one

teaspoon of cocoa powder, two teaspoons of gingerbread spices, one tablespoon of cornflour, four eggs, one orange, a pinch of salt, 100 g of hazelnuts, 50 g of sugar, 80 g of water.

And here's how it works:
Knead cocoa powder, gingerbread spice, salt, flour, butter, brown sugar and form a dough ball. Store this dough ball in the fridge for about 30 minutes. Now bake the cake base blind. Line a springform pan with baking paper. Roll out the dough on a work surface and line the edge of the springform pan about 3 cm high. Cover this dough again with baking parchment and place dry pulses on top, then bake at approx. 180°C for 15 minutes. For the mixture, mix cornflour, vanilla pod pulp, maple syrup, ricotta, eggs, juice and orange peel. Pour this mixture onto the pre-baked base and bake at approx. 160°C for 40 minutes.

For the hazelnut caramel, coarsely grind the hazelnuts in a mortar and boil them up with 80 g of water and the 50 g of sugar until the sugar caramelises.

10.12.3 Cheesecake Tiramisu in a glass
You need:
60 g of butter, 120 g of ladyfingers, 30 g of espresso powder (instant), 60g of dark chocolate, 450 g of low-fat curd cheese, 550 g of mascarpone, 100 g of whipped

cream, 170 g of erythritol, 20 g of vanilla sugar, five eggs, 20 g of starch or custard powder.

And here's how it works:

Melt the butter. Put three pieces of the ladyfingers aside, crumble the rest. Mix the butter and the crumbs, place them in six small ovenproof dishes and press them well on the bottom. Preheat the oven to 150°C. Make the cream. Mix the espresso, finely grated chocolate, quark, mascarpone, cream, erythritol, vanilla sugar, eggs and starch until smooth. Pour this mixture into the six moulds, place in a suitably large pot and pour hot water up to 1 cm below the rim. Cook in the oven for about 45 minutes. Let it cool down. Coarsely divide the rest of the lady fingers and sprinkle them on the moulds.

10.12.4 Pear-Rhubarb Crumble

You need:

350 g of pears, for example Williams Christ, 280 g of rhubarb, three tablespoons of erythritol, juice and grated lemon, one tablespoon of custard powder, 40 g of almond biscuits, 30 g of butter, 30 g of oat flakes, two packs of vanilla sugar.

And here's how it works:

Wash the pears, quarter them, remove the seeds and cut them into pieces. Clean the rhubarb and cut into 2 cm thick pieces. Put pears and rhubarb in a pot, add erythritol and lemon juice and bring it to the boil covered. Mix the vanilla custard powder with two tablespoons of water to bind the pear-rhubarb mixture, bring to the boil and set aside. Pour the compote into small glasses.

Coarsely chop the almond biscuits with a knife. Melt the butter in a pan. Fry the oat flakes and almond biscuits in the pan until golden brown. Sprinkle with a little icing sugar and let them caramelise. Put the cooled almond biscuits Oatmeal Crumble on the compote and serve.

10.12.5 Warm chocolate cake

You need:
110 g of dark chocolate, 70 g of butter, 50 g of erythritol, a pinch of salt, two eggs, 20 g of flour.
And here's how it works:
Preheat the oven to 170 °C. Grease four small ovenproof baking pans with butter and sprinkle with flour. Melt the chocolate in a hot water bath. Beat the soft butter, erythritol and a pinch of salt in a bowl with a hand mixer until foamy. Add the eggs one by one and continue beating. Stir in the liquid chocolate. Add the flour and stir in with a wooden spoon. Pour the dough evenly into the moulds and bake in the oven for about ten minutes. Serve the warm chocolate cake on a small plate, for example with a fruit sauce and sprinkle with icing sugar.

10.12.6 Semolina crème brulée with mango

You need:

Half a mango, 500 g of milk 3.5%, a pinch of salt, 60 g of erythritol, the pulp of a vanilla pod, 50 g of wheat semolina, 40 g of brown sugar.

And here's how it works:

Cut a mango in half, remove the flesh and cut into cubes. Bring milk and sugar together with a pinch of salt to the boil. Add half of the mango to the mixture and puree everything using a blender. Stir in wheat semolina with a whisk. Let it swell for a short time and fill it into fireproof glasses while still warm. Divide the remaining mango between the glasses, sprinkle with brown sugar and caramelise with a gas burner.

10.12.7 Carrots cup cake with walnuts

You need:

150 g of carrots, 150 g of walnuts, 50 g of wheat flour, 140 g of erythritol, three eggs.

And here's how it works:

Wash and peel the carrots. Grate finely on a kitchen grater. Separate the yolks from the egg white. Add 100 g of erythritol to the yolks. Then mix with a hand mixer until foamy. Beat the egg white with 40 g of erythritol and a pinch of salt until stiff. Finely chop the walnuts. Carefully mix the egg yolks and the egg white mixture together and fold in the walnuts, flour and carrots.

Grease four ovenproof baking dishes with butter and sprinkle with flour or breadcrumbs. Pour in the carrot mixture and bake at 180°C for about 45 minutes. Sprinkle with icing sugar before serving.

10.12.8 Rhubarb Crumble

You need:

190 g of erythritol, 90 g of butter, 610 g of rhubarb, a vanilla pod, juice and rind of one lemon, 70 g of oat flakes, 80 g of flour, one orange.

And here's how it works:

Mix the oat flakes, a pinch of salt, flour and erythritol. Add butter in small pieces and knead until small lumps are formed. Wash and clean the rhubarb and cut it into pieces about 2 cm long. Halve the vanilla pod and scrape out the pulp. Wash the orange and rub the skin off. Mix the rhubarb, erythritol, lemon juice, vanilla pulp, orange peel and leave it to stand for about five minutes. Pour the rhubarb mixture into a small casserole dish and spread the crumbles over it. Bake in a preheated oven at 210°C for approx. 40 minutes. A scoop of vanilla ice cream goes perfectly with this. Serve hot.

10.12.9 Low Carb cream cheese pancakes

You need:

35 g of cream cheese, one egg, 50 g of almond flour, a teaspoon of xylitol, a pinch of salt, a teaspoon of coconut oil, 60 g of almond milk.

And here's how it works:

Mix all ingredients in a suitable container. The dough should not be too thick. Add some of the almond milk. Put the pancakes in a pan with a little oil as usual, until golden. Goes well with berries or vanilla ice cream.

Xylitol (chemically pentanentol) belongs to the group of sugar alcohols and is used, for example, in dental care chewing gums. Xylitol is similar in taste to normal household sugar, has almost the same sweetening power, but only one third of the calories. Almond flour can be used similarly to wheat flour, but the amount of calories is reduced by about 53%.

10.12.10 Vanilla-Ricotta cream with blueberries

You need:

250 g of ricotta, half a vanilla pod, juice of one lemon, 50 g of erythritol, 250 g of blueberries, half a bunch of lemon balm, some icing sugar.

And here's how it works:

Place the ricotta in a bowl. Cut the vanilla pod lengthwise and scrape out the pulp. Add the vanilla pulp, juice and zest of one lemon, 50 g of erythritol and a pinch of salt to the ricotta. Wash the blueberries. Pluck the lemon balm, add it to the blueberries with the icing sugar and mix.

Ricotta is an Italian cream cheese that can be made from sheep or cow's milk. Translated, ricotta means „cooked again". Alternatively, cottage cheese can be used, which tastes just as mild. Also similar to ricotta is the Indian Panir cheese.

10.13 Baking

10.13.1 Best rye mixed bread without sourdough

You need:

345 g of wheat flour type 550, 110 g of rye flour, two teaspoons of salt, half a cube of fresh yeast, 360 g of water at room temperature, salt without anti-caking agent and not iodised.

And here's how it works:

Mix all ingredients in a large bowl and then cover. Let it rest for at least 16 hours, preferably in a warm, dark place. The dough should now have gained considerable volume. Carefully place the dough on a work surface sprinkled with flour and, without destroying its volume, knead it carefully once again. Let the dough rest again for two hours, covered with a towel. Preheat the oven to 230° C, put a bowl of water in the bottom of the oven. Place the dough on a baking tray covered with baking paper. If you have a cast-iron roaster with a lid, you can also use it. In this case, bake the first 20 minutes with the lid on, the rest of the time without the lid.

10.13.2 Wholemeal spelt bread without rising

You need:

500 g of wholemeal spelt flour, approx. 120 g of grains of your choice, for example pumpkin seeds, sunflower seeds or walnut kernels, half a tablespoon of rock salt, half a

litre of warm water, a cube of yeast, two tablespoons of apple vinegar.

And here's how it works:

Roast the grains in a pan without fat. Pour the warm water into a large bowl, mix the cube of yeast, salt and apple vinegar. Add the grains. Add the wholemeal spelt flour and mix well with a mixing spoon. Line a box form with baking paper. Add the bread dough. The oven does not need to be preheated. Then put the box form in the oven and bake at 190° C for one hour.

10.13.3 Foccacia

You need:

1 cube of fresh yeast, 200 ml of lukewarm whole milk, 20g of erythritol, 70g of pine nuts, 70 g of black olives pitted, 130 g of dried tomatoes pickled in oil, 500 g of flour type 405, salt, one egg, 3 tbsp of tomato paste, 2 tsp of dried oregano, 450 g of cherry tomatoes, two sprigs of rosemary, coarse rock salt.

And here's how it works:

Mix lukewarm milk, yeast and sugar. Roast the pine nuts in a pan without fat. Let cool and chop. Cut the olives into quarters. Drain dried tomatoes and collect oil. Set aside 100 ml of tomato oil. Dice the tomatoes. Mix the flour, pinch of salt and the yeast mixture. Add the oil, dried tomatoes and the egg. Knead into a smooth dough. Knead in the tomato paste, pine nuts, dried tomatoes, olives and oregano. Leave the dough to rise in a warm place, covered, for at least two hours. Preheat the oven to 180° C Form the dough into a large flat cake and spread it flat on a baking paper. Press depressions into the dough. Wash and dry the tomatoes and spread them in the depressions. Wash, dry and pluck the rosemary and spread it on the dough. Sprinkle everything with rock salt and bake in the oven for approx. 30-35 minutes.

11. List of recipes

Alkaline diet	93
Antipasti with vegetables, mushrooms and olives	140
Apple and horseradish soup	107
Arancini - Sicilian rice balls	152
Asparagus Fennel Salad	103
Asparagus ham salad with couscous	88
Asparagus salad—gnocchi—wild garlic pesto	91
Avocado-Banana-Apple Smoothie	130
Baked aubergine and carrots	144
Baked aubergine, celery puree, carrots	149
Baking	162
Bami Goreng with broccoli and tempeh	146
Beetroot sweet potato soup	106
Best rye mixed bread without sourdough	162
Birch muesli with carrot boscoop salad	135
Blueberry pumpernickel dressing	125
Braised meatballs	142
Bulgur salad with feta and beetroot	89
Buttermilk-blackberry dressing	122
Carrot soup with spelt croutons	113
Carrots cup cake with walnuts	158
Cheesecake Tiramisu in a glass	155
Chiapudding	104
Chick peas smoothie, Greek yoghurt and broccoli	130
Chicken Feta Broccoli Casserole	99
Chickpea salad—smoked salmon strips	86
Chinese Cabbage Blueberry Smoothie	127
Chorizo stew	110
Coffee Cream	154
Corn salad—feta cheese	87
Courgette spaghetti with lentil bolognese	148

Cranberry and hazelnut dressing	123
Curry lentil soup with baked cauliflower	108
Foccacia	163
French onion soup	111
Fried cod on courgette vegetables	96
Fried fillet of gilthead	138
Gazpacho—cold tomato soup	103
Ginger Grape Carrot Smoothie	131
Green Detox Smoothie	128
Grilled Bread	138
Grilled vegetables with rocket salad	94
Healthy breakfast	134
Keto recipes	96
Ketogenic almond bread	98
Kohlrabi Savoy Soup	117
Konjac noodles with avocadopesto	97
Leek-Paprika Muffin	151
Lentil roasts	96
Lentil soup with chard and minced meat	116
Lentil soup with spinach	112
Low Carb cream cheese pancake	159
Mango-Jalapeño Dressing	124
Mediterranean	138
Melon Granite	95
Minestrone	111
Oatmeal with maple syrup and banana	136
Orange bread salad—chicken breast fillets	92
Oven vegetables	93
Pak Choi with ginger-garlic sauce and sesame	145
Pan of vegetables with Thai asparagus	100
Panzanella (Italian bread salad)	90
Parsley root soup	114
Pasta salad with mozzarella	141
Pea and balm dressing	124

Pear-Rhubarb Crumble	156
Penne in tuna tomato sauce	140
Pineapple-Mango Detox Smoothie	132
Potato and mushroom soup	109
Pumpkin and Spinach Curry	101
Pumpkin and turnip soup	105
Radish potato salad	90
Radish spaghetti with vegetable bolognese	99
Raw food	103
Recipes	86
Rhubarb Crumble	159
Ricotta cheesecake - hazelnut caramel	154
Ricotta Quiche	98
Salad dressings	120
Salads & Bowls	86
Sauerkraut-Grapefruit Smoothie	129
Semolina crème brulée with mango	158
Skyr with seeds, oranges and banana	134
Smoothie	127
Snacks	151
Soups	105
Spanish potato salad - olives - thyme	88
Spelt bread with avocado cream and graved salmon	134
Spicy noodle soup with chicken	118
Spinach and savoy cabbage smoothie with pear	131
Spinach Crostini au gratin	152
Sweet potato, chickpeas and almond sauce	147
Sweet reward	154
Thai coconut soup with rice noodles	106
Tomatoes stuffed with oriental couscous	146
Turnips Potato soup with wild garlic Pesto	115
Vanilla-Ricotta cream with blueberries	160
Vegan dishes	144
Vinaigrette, classic	120

Warm chocolate cake   157
Wasabi lime dressing   121
Wholemeal spelt bread without rising   162
Wild herb soup   93
Yoghurt dressing   121

12. Conclusion

Losing weight healthily is a big challenge for many people. If it were easy, there would be no overweight people. Unfortunately, the reality looks different for many of us. It takes discipline and perseverance to stick to a change in diet, and it takes determination to defeat your inner bastard. But if you prepare yourself properly and choose a path that you can cope with, you will achieve your goal. While reading this book, you were able to deal intensively with the subject of nutrition, change of diet and motivation. The nutritional recommendations in this book, your mindset and your ability to overcome your inner bastard are the three most important pillars for a successful change of diet. So from now on, if you are aiming for a new life with a different diet, you will be well prepared.

Which shape you finally decide on is entirely up to you. It is important that it adapts to your life and not the other way round. It is important that you don't have to change your life seriously, because this way it is usually easier to make the change and you don't feel so restricted. Take this book to heart and internalise the principles presented here. You will certainly succeed in switching to a healthy diet, and you will be able to lose weight and maintain your weight without succumbing to the yo-yo effect.

13. Feedback

I am happy about your feedback. Did you like the book? Then I would be very happy about a fair evaluation. Just click on the following link.

https://amzn.to/3nASlrW

Many thanks for your support!

Did you not like the book? Even then I am very happy about every feedback. Honest feedback is essential for me to improve myself. So if you have any suggestions or ideas for improvement, and also if you want to give your displeasure some breathing space, I would be very happy to receive a mail. You can send any kind of request to the following e-mail address: book_manufacture@outlook.com.

Thank you very much for your support in this case as well!

Best regards
Liam Wade

14. Sources

[1] https://www.timsquirrell.com/blog/2017/2/17/thoughts-on-paleo-evolutionary-nutrition-and-falsification

[2] http://www.getbritainstanding.org/health-risks.php

[3] https://www.heartuk.org.uk/genetic-conditions/metabolic-syndrome

[4] https://www.nhs.uk/conditions/type-2-diabetes/

[5] https://www.diabetes.co.uk/diabetes-types.html

[6] https://thehealthsciencesacademy.org/health-tips/is-sugar-an-addictive-drug/

[7] https://scienceblog.cancerresearchuk.org/2017/05/15/sugar-and-cancer-what-you-need-to-know/

[8] https://www.diabetes.co.uk/body/visceral-fat.html

[9] https://peacefuleating.co.uk/ideal-weight-healthy-weight-natural-weight-happy-weight/

[10] https://www.nhs.uk/live-well/healthy-weight/bmi-calculator/

[11] https://www.frontiersin.org/articles/10.3389/fpsyg.2019.01221/full

[12] https://www.goodtoknow.co.uk/wellbeing/mediterranean-diet-65356

[13] https://www.netdoctor.co.uk/healthy-eating/a10842/fibre/

[14] https://www.eufic.org/en/whats-in-food/article/dietary-fibre-whats-its-role-in-a-healthy-diet

[15] https://www.drmyhill.co.uk/wiki/Ketogenic_diet_-_a_connection_between_mitochondria_and_diet

16   https://www.frontiersin.org/articles/10.3389/fphar.2018.01162/full

17   https://www.bbc.co.uk/food/articles/what_should_you_eat_for_a_healthy_gut

18   https://graziadaily.co.uk/life/food-and-drink/alkaline-diet/

19   https://www.bimuno.com/news/what-are-fermented-foods-and-why-are-they-so-popular/

20   https://www.bda.uk.com/resource/fermented-foods.html

21   https://www.independent.co.uk/life-style/food-and-drink/features/what-happens-your-body-hour-after-eating-sugar-a6879026.html

22   https://www.motionnutrition.com/spot-avoid-hidden-sugars/

2 http://www.getbritainstanding.org/health-risks.php

3 https://www.heartuk.org.uk/genetic-conditions/metabolic-syndrome

4 https://www.nhs.uk/conditions/type-2-diabetes/

5 https://www.diabetes.co.uk/diabetes-types.html

6 https://thehealthsciencesacademy.org/health-tips/is-sugar-an-addictive-drug/

7 https://scienceblog.cancerresearchuk.org/2017/05/15/sugar-and-cancer-what-you-need-to-know/

[8] https://www.diabetes.co.uk/body/visceral-fat.html

[9] https://peacefuleating.co.uk/ideal-weight-healthy-weight-natural-weight-happy-weight/

[10] https://www.nhs.uk/live-well/healthy-weight/bmi-calculator/

[11] https://www.frontiersin.org/articles/10.3389/fpsyg.2019.01221/full

[12] https://www.goodtoknow.co.uk/wellbeing/mediterranean-diet-65356

[13] https://www.netdoctor.co.uk/healthy-eating/a10842/fibre/

[14] https://www.eufic.org/en/whats-in-food/article/dietary-fibre-whats-its-role-in-a-healthy-diet

[15] https://www.drmyhill.co.uk/wiki/Ketogenic_diet_-_a_connection_between_mitochondria_and_diet

[16] https://www.frontiersin.org/articles/10.3389/fphar.2018.01162/full

[17] https://www.bbc.co.uk/food/articles/what_should_you_eat_for_a_healthy_gut

[18] https://graziadaily.co.uk/life/food-and-drink/alkaline-diet/

[19] https://www.bimuno.com/news/what-are-fermented-foods-and-why-are-they-so-popular/

[20] https://www.bda.uk.com/resource/fermented-foods.html

[21] https://www.independent.co.uk/life-style/food-and-drink/features/what-happens-your-body-hour-after-eating-sugar-a6879026.html

[22] https://www.motionnutrition.com/spot-avoid-hidden-sugars/

15. Copyright

16. Disclaimer

The implementation of all information, instructions and strategies contained in this book is at your own risk. The author cannot be held liable for any damages of any kind for any legal reason. Liability claims against the author for material or non-material damage caused by the use or non-use of the information or by the use of incorrect and/or incomplete information are excluded in principle. Any legal and compensation claims are therefore excluded. This work has been compiled and written down with the greatest care and to the best of our knowledge and belief. However, the author accepts no responsibility for the topicality, completeness and quality of the information. Nor can printing errors and misinformation be completely excluded. No legal responsibility or liability of any kind can be assumed for incorrect information provided by the author.

17. Liability for links

My books contain links to external websites of third parties, over whose contents we have no influence. Therefore I cannot take any responsibility for these external contents. The respective provider or operator of the sites is always responsible for the contents of the linked sites. The linked pages were checked for possible legal violations at the time of linking. Illegal contents were not recognisable at the time of linking.

However, a permanent control of the contents of the linked pages is not reasonable without concrete evidence of a violation of the law. If I become aware of any infringements, I will remove such links immediately.

18. Imprint

Contact us: Andreas Löw, Fünfhausenstraße 24a, 31832 Springe, Germany
book_manufacture@outlook.com
Keyword: eat yourself slim

Cover: Depositphotos_114782712_ds

Printed in Great Britain
by Amazon

61092001R00102